Your Child with Inflammatory Bowel Disease

A Johns Hopkins Press Health Book

Your Child with Inflammatory Bowel Disease

A Family Guide for Caregiving

North American Society for Pediatric Gastroenterology, Hepatology and Nutrition

EDITORS-IN-CHIEF
Maria Oliva-Hemker, M.D.
David Ziring, M.D.
Athos Bousvaros, M.D.

The Johns Hopkins University Press
Baltimore

The Johns Hopkins University Press
2715 North Charles Street
Baltimore, Maryland 21218-4363
www.press.jhu.edu

ISBN-13: 978-0-8018-9555-5 (hardcover)
ISBN-10: 0-8018-9555-3 (hardcover)
ISBN-13: 978-0-8018-9556-2 (paperback)
ISBN-10: 0-8018-9556-1 (paperback)

Illustrations on pages 5, 6, 8, 12, 14, 22, 26, 37, 38, 49, 51, 83, 129, 131, 136, 169, 174
by Jacqueline Schaffer
Illustrations on pages 21, 47, 59, 65, 78, 90, 159, 163, 185, 195, 198, 203, 219
by Susanna Natti

Special discounts are available for bulk purchases of this book. For more information,
please contact Special Sales at 410-516-6936 or specialsales@press.jhu.edu.

The Johns Hopkins University Press uses environmentally friendly book materials,
including recycled text paper that is composed of at least 30 percent post-consumer
waste, whenever possible. All of our book papers are acid-free, and our jackets and
covers are printed on paper with recycled content.

❧ Contents

🦋 Contributors

Susan S. Baker, M.D., Ph.D.
Children's Hospital of Buffalo
Buffalo, New York

Robert N. Baldassano, M.D.*
Children's Hospital of Philadelphia
Philadelphia, Pennsylvania

Keith J. Benkov, M.D.*
Mt. Sinai Medical Center
New York, New York

Athos Bousvaros, M.D.
Children's Hospital
Boston, Massachusetts

Jeffrey B. Brown, M.D.
Children's Memorial Hospital
Chicago, Illinois

Steven Brown, M.B.B.S., Ph.D.
Mount Sinai School of Medicine
New York, New York

Mitchell B. Cohen, M.D.
Cincinnati Children's Hospital
Medical Center
Cincinnati, Ohio

Stanley A. Cohen, M.D.
Children's Center for Digestive
Healthcare
Atlanta, Georgia

Richard B. Colletti, M.D.
University of Vermont
Burlington, Vermont

Wallace V. Crandall, M.D.
Nationwide Children's Hospital
Columbus, Ohio

Karen Denise Crissinger, M.D., Ph.D.
University of South Alabama
Mobile, Alabama

Fredric Daum, M.D.
Winthrop University Hospital
New York, New York

Marla Dubinsky, M.D.
Cedars-Sinai Medical Center
Los Angeles, California

Adi R. Ferrara**
Bellevue, Washington

George D. Ferry, M.D.
Texas Children's Hospital
Houston, Texas

Benjamin Gold, M.D.
Children's Center for Digestive
Healthcare
Atlanta, Georgia

Anne M. Griffiths, M.D.*
Hospital for Sick Children
Toronto, Ontario, Canada

Sandeep Gupta, M.D.
Riley Hospital for Children
Indianapolis, Indiana

Melvin B. Heyman, M.D., M.P.H.
San Francisco Children's Hospital
San Francisco, California

Leslie M. Higuchi, M.D.
Children's Hospital
Boston, Massachusetts

Jeffrey S. Hyams, M.D.*
Connecticut Children's Medical
  Center
Hartford, Connecticut

Mark J. Integlia, M.D.
Cape Elizabeth, Maine

David M. Israel, M.D., F.R.C.P.
British Columbia Children's
  Hospital
Vancouver, British Columbia,
  Canada

Esther Israel, M.D.
Massachusetts General Hospital
Boston, Massachusetts

Robert M. Issenman, M.D.
McMaster Children's Hospital
Hamilton, Ontario, Canada

Howard A. Kader, M.D.
Sinai Hospital of Baltimore
Baltimore, Maryland

Marsha Kay, M.D.
Cleveland Clinic Foundation
Cleveland, Ohio

David J. Keljo, M.D., Ph.D.
University of Pittsburgh
  School of Medicine
Pittsburgh, Pennsylvania

Barbara S. Kirschner, M.D.
University of Chicago Children's
  Hospital
Chicago, Illinois

Alan M. Leichtner, M.D.
Children's Hospital
Boston, Massachusetts

David R. Mack, M.D.
Children's Hospital of Eastern
  Ontario
Ottawa, Ontario, Canada

Laura Mackner
Nationwide Children's Hospital
Columbus, Ohio

Lori Mahajan, M.D.
Cleveland Clinic Foundation
Cleveland, Ohio

Petar Mamula, M.D.
Children's Hospital of Philadelphia
Philadelphia, Pennsylvania

James F. Markowitz, M.D.*
North Shore–LIJ Health System
New Hyde Park, New York

Jonathan E. Markowitz, M.D.
Greenville Children's Hospital
Greenville, South Carolina

Adelina McDuffie, R.N., M.S.,
C.P.N.P.
Children's Hospital of Kings
  Daughters
Norfolk, Virginia

Mary Susan Moyer, M.D.
Cincinnati Children's Hospital
  Medical Center
Cincinnati, Ohio

Maria Oliva-Hemker, M.D.
The Johns Hopkins Hospital
Baltimore, Maryland

Anthony Otley, M.D.
IWK Health Centre
Halifax, Nova Scotia, Canada

Susan Peck, R.N., M.S.N., C.P.N.P.
Children's Hospital of Philadelphia
Philadelphia, Pennsylvania

David A. Piccoli, M.D.
Children's Hospital of Philadelphia
Philadelphia, Pennsylvania

D. Brent Polk, M.D.
Vanderbilt University School of
Medicine
Nashville, Tennessee

Joel R. Rosh, M.D.
Morristown Memorial Hospital
Morristown, New Jersey

Gary J. Russell, M.D.
Massachusetts General Hospital
Boston, Massachusetts

Bruce Sands, M.D.
Massacusetts General Hospital
Boston, Massachusetts

Judy B. Splawski, M.D.
Rainbow Babies and Children's
Hospital
Cleveland, Ohio

Maya D. Srivastava, M.D., Ph.D.
Philadelphia, Pennsylvania
Cleveland, Ohio

Michael C. Stephens, M.D.
Medical College of Wisconsin
Milwaukee, Wisconsin

Francisco Sylvester, M.D.
Connecticut Childrens Medical
Center
Hartford, Connecticut

Eva Szigethy, M.D.
University of Pittsburgh
Pittsburgh, Pennsylvania

Vasundhara Tolia, M.D.
Children's Hospital of Michigan
Detroit, Michigan

William R. Treem, M.D.
Children's Hospital at Downstate
Brooklyn, New York

John N. Udall, Jr., M.D., Ph.D.
West Virginia University
Charleston, West Virginia

Eric Vasiliauskas, M.D.
Cedars-Sinai Medical Center
Los Angeles, California

Menno Verhave, M.D.
Children's Hospital
Boston, Massachusetts

Steven L. Werlin, M.D.
Medical College of Wisconsin
Milwaukee, Wisconsin

Harland S. Winter, M.D.*
Massacusetts General Hospital
for Children
Boston, Massachusetts

Robert Wyllie, M.D.
Cleveland Clinic Foundation
Cleveland, Ohio

David Ziring, M.D.
University of California
Los Angeles, California

* Founding Editor
** Medical Writer and Editor

❧   Preface

The first time I heard the phrase "Crohn disease" I was about 5 years old. I didn't know what it was, but I knew this: Crohn disease was the reason my mom was in the hospital and not home with me. Crohn disease took on an entirely new meaning when I was diagnosed with the disease myself, when I was 13 years old. A curious soul even then, I bombarded my doctors with questions about my new diagnosis:

Was I going to have to be in the hospital like my mom?
Would I have this disease forever?
How did I get Crohn disease?

Their answers only fueled my curiosity. I needed to understand more. I can't be positive, but I am fairly certain that my diagnosis of Crohn disease led me to medical school and, eventually, to become a pediatric gastroenterologist.

Information about inflammatory bowel disease (IBD) is very important to me, and I make patient education a mainstay of my practice. I have even been known to quiz my patients in the office. Understanding what symptoms mean, why things happen, and how medications work is important. I believe that the more patients and families understand these issues, the more likely they are to take their medications and to seek help early when problems develop.

My knowledge of IBD has grown exponentially since I was first diagnosed. I have learned from my own experience as a patient and as a physician, and I continue to learn from the patients I take care of. I have learned that no person's illness is exactly the same as another person's. And I have learned that despite my best efforts, I can't always tell what is important to a patient's particular case.

While I wouldn't wish the diagnosis of IBD on anyone, I can honestly say that Crohn disease has made me a better person. I have learned perspective. I now know what's important. I have had the privilege of watching children with IBD grow up and follow their dreams. I have met architects, teachers, firefighters, a professional golfer, a NASCAR driver, and countless other people with IBD. I have learned that having IBD isn't fun, but that it doesn't stop you from succeeding at anything you set your mind to.

This book is not a substitute for talking with your doctor or your child's doctor, but it is nevertheless a wonderful resource. It provides reliable information that can help satisfy curiosity as well as explain the importance of symptoms, the role of tests and operations, and the actions and side effects of medications. It can help you to take better care of your child or yourself by making you a better partner with your child's doctor or your own doctor to meet the challenges of these diseases. My family and I would have appreciated having the insight and resources found in this book throughout our experience of living with IBD.

Cheryl Blank, D.O.
Pediatric Gastroenterologist and Inflammatory Bowel Disease Specialist
Maine Medical Center, Portland, Maine

Acknowledgments

This book reflects the hard work of more than fifty experts, each of whom wrote a section of the book that was then integrated into the whole. The project was started several years ago by a team of physicians who solicited contributions from members of the North American Society for Pediatric Gastroenterology, Hepatology and Nutrition. Those physicians are designated as "founding editors" (with an asterisk) in the List of Contributors. The manuscript was revised by Adi Ferrara, a medical writer. The physicians who became the editors-in-chief then updated the content, added new sections, and rewrote the book extensively to give it one voice. The final revising, editing, and addition of illustrations were performed by the wonderful team at the Johns Hopkins University Press.

Because this book has been extensively rewritten, we cannot assign authorship of a specific chapter to any individual or group of individuals. This book should therefore be considered a group effort by all the people listed as contributing authors. If we have inadvertently omitted any contributor during this process, we apologize.

We would like to dedicate this book to the memory of Susan Moyer, a caring and kind physician who spent her life improving the health of children with Crohn disease and ulcerative colitis.

Publication of this book was made possible by an independent educational grant from Shire.

Part I

Introduction to IBD

🐝 1
An Overview of Inflammatory Bowel Disease

Starting Out

If you are reading this book, it's likely that your child has been diagnosed with a form of inflammatory bowel disease. If your child has been diagnosed recently, a number of questions may be running through your mind:

Why does my child have this condition? What caused it?
Is it serious?
How is it treated?
What should my child eat?

This section of the book describes the healthy digestive system, and it describes how inflammatory bowel disease causes digestive problems. Later chapters in the book will answer many of the other questions you may have. You will probably have still more questions after reading this book; if you do, the resources listed in the back of the book may help. Don't forget, though, that your health care team should be your primary source for medical knowledge about your child's illness.

What Is IBD?

Inflammatory bowel disease (IBD) is a general term that usually refers to one of three different conditions: Crohn disease (CD), ulcerative colitis (UC), and indeterminate colitis (IC). Crohn disease used to be called Crohn's disease and sometimes still is. Indeterminate colitis is a term used to describe IBD when physicians cannot determine whether the person has Crohn disease or ulcerative colitis, though a diagnosis of one or the other often becomes clearer over time.

Crohn disease and ulcerative colitis are different genetically, they affect different portions of the intestine, and they are treated differently. However, CD and UC share enough features to group them both under the name "inflammatory bowel disease." IBD causes inflammation (swelling and irritation) somewhere in the digestive system, most commonly in the large intestine (the *colon*). IBD can also cause problems outside the digestive system.

The inflammation of IBD occurs when a person's immune cells attack the person's own digestive system (the gastrointestinal, or GI, tract). The immune cells are the cells that normally clear bacteria and other disease-causing organisms from the body. Why does the body attack its own GI tract? Research suggests that IBD occurs when a person who inherits genes that make him susceptible to IBD is exposed to something in the environment that makes his intestine's immune system react against the bowel (see figure 1.1). When inflammation occurs, the intestine becomes red and swollen.

Researchers have not yet isolated all the genes involved in Crohn disease or ulcerative colitis. They have also not discovered which specific environmental factors trigger the disease. However, research into inheritance and environment has made great progress in the past twenty years. Physicians and scientists hope that with ongoing research, we will be able to identify the causes of CD and UC. Research is continuing in these areas.

We return to the discussion of ulcerative colitis and Crohn disease near the end of this chapter. First, though, we briefly review the structure and functions of the GI tract and explore why the intestine is so important to human health, what *inflammation* means, and what happens when the intestine becomes inflamed.

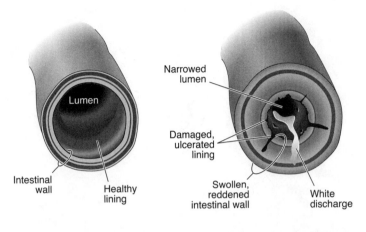

Normal small intestine   **Inflamed small intestine in CD**

Figure 1.1. Cross-sectional views of normal and inflamed small intestine. The intestine looks like a hollow tube. Food and liquid pass through the center of the tube (the intestinal lumen). As nutrients pass, they are broken down and absorbed on the inner surface of the intestine (the mucosa, or inner lining). The wall of the intestine is normally thin (*left*). When the intestine is inflamed, as in Crohn disease (*right*), the wall of the intestine becomes thickened and red, and the lumen may become narrow.

What Is the Gastrointestinal Tract, and What Does It Do?

Structure and Functions of the Digestive System

The primary role of the gastrointestinal tract (or digestive system) is to convert food into simple substances that can be used as energy. Food is composed of three main substances: carbohydrates (sugars and starches), proteins, and fats (lipids). The digestive system takes food, grinds it, and breaks it down into "building blocks," including simple sugars, amino acids, and fatty acids. These building blocks can be absorbed by intestinal cells, delivered to the bloodstream, and used by the different organs of the body, including the heart, lungs, brain,

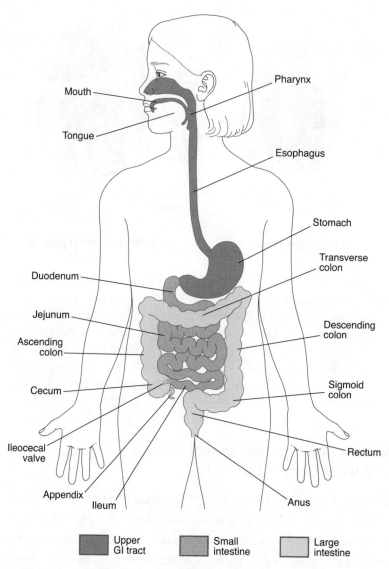

Mouth

Tongue

Pharynx

Esophagus

Stomach

Transverse colon

Duodenum

Jejunum

Ascending colon

Cecum

Descending colon

Sigmoid colon

Ileocecal valve

Rectum

Appendix

Ileum

Anus

Upper GI tract

Small intestine

Large intestine

Figure 1.2. Map of the digestive system. Food starts in the mouth, passes through the esophagus, then into the stomach and the first part of the small intestine (duodenum). The upper part of the small intestine is the jejunum, and the lower part is the ileum. Digested intestinal contents leaving the small intestine enter the first part of the large intestine, or cecum. They then pass through the ascending colon, transverse colon, descending colon, sigmoid colon, and rectum before being expelled.

and muscles. If the intestine doesn't function properly, the body can't digest food well, and the person is at risk of developing malnutrition (lack of calories and energy).

The gastrointestinal tract consists of different segments (figure 1.2). The mouth and *pharynx* (throat) swallow food and deliver it to the esophagus, a long tube that carries food from the mouth to the stomach. The stomach is a powerful muscle whose main purpose is to mechanically grind food into small pieces (food particles). Once the food particles are sufficiently small, they pass into the small intestine. The small intestine can be thought of as a very long, flexible tube or cylinder—in the average adult, the length of the small intestine is approximately 18 to 20 feet. The inner portion of the cylinder, where food, fluid, and digestive juices are located, is called the *lumen*.

The main purpose of the small intestine is to absorb food and water. Once food particles enter the small intestine, the particles mix with intestinal fluid and digestive juices from the liver and pancreas. Here, in the intestinal lumen, foods are broken down into their building blocks. Specifically, starches are broken down into simple sugars, proteins are broken down into amino acids, and fats are broken down into fatty acids and *monoglycerides*. At this point, foods are ready to be absorbed by the small intestinal lining (*intestinal epithelium*).

The cells of the small intestinal lining can be seen only with a microscope. The most common cell in the intestinal lining is the intestinal absorptive cell (the *enterocyte*); billions of these cells line the intestine. They are specially designed to transport the nutritional building blocks (sugars, amino acids, and fatty acids) into the bloodstream. To improve digestion, these cells are positioned in fingerlike projections called *villi*. Thus, the inner surface of the small intestine is not flat but is composed of thousands and thousands of little "intestinal fingers" that help absorb food. Healthy villi can be seen by the gastroenterologist with a high-magnification endoscope or under the microscope (figure 1.3).

The small intestine gradually pushes food particles down the length of its 18 or so feet to the *ileocecal valve* (the valve that connects

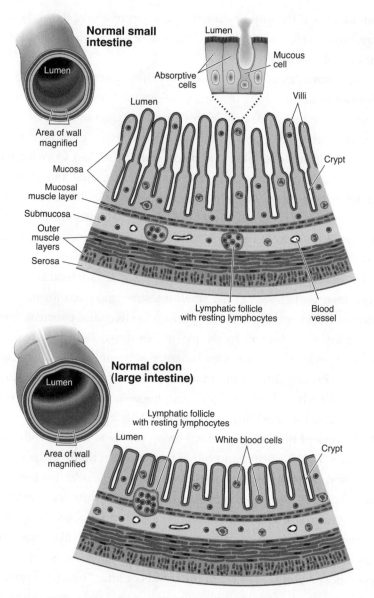

Figure 1.3. Magnified views of the lining of the small intestine and the colon, showing villi and immune system cells. In the small intestine, the absorptive and mucous cells lining the inner layer (*inset, top*) are arranged in fingerlike structures called villi. The villi help increase surface area for absorption of food. Below the villi are crypts, which secrete intestinal fluid. Underneath the in-

the small intestine and the large intestine). By the time food particles leave the small intestine, most of their nutritional value has been extracted, and what is left is undigested food (roughage). What enters the large intestine (colon) is a mushy brown fluid. The main role of the large intestine is to further thicken the stool by absorbing water from the stool into the body. Thus, the stool that comes out of the anus is usually formed. Although the colon is useful in preventing dehydration, one does not need the colon to absorb food, and people can maintain their weight and hydration without a colon, as long as they eat and drink enough.

The Intestine's Immune System

Another role of the intestine is to protect against infections. Every day, the intestine is exposed to "invaders" from outside our bodies. These invaders include the bacteria and viruses we swallow after inhaling them through our nose, bacteria in the soil and ground, and the organisms that live in contaminated food and drinking water. To protect from infection, the intestine has an elaborate immune system. This system is not an organ like the heart or gut but a collective name for cells that travel around the body. The best known cells of the immune system are the white blood cells, which can be found both in the blood and in the tissues (for example, the lungs and the gut). These immune system cells (white blood cells and others) live in the different layers of the intestine. The main purpose of the intestine's immune system is to prevent bacteria and viruses from entering the bloodstream and doing damage throughout the body. If the cells of the im-

---

nermost layer (mucosa) is another layer (submucosa) that includes blood vessels (for absorption of digested nutrients) and cells of the immune system (lymphatic follicles). Underneath the mucosa and submucosa are muscle layers that can contract and push food through the intestine.

The colon (large intestine) has a structure similar to the structure of the small intestine. However, because the colon is not as important as the small intestine in absorbing digested food and nutrients, its surface is flat, without villi.

mune system are inappropriately turned on, or *activated*, however, they have the potential to damage the person's own intestine.

What Does *Inflammation* Mean?

The word *inflammation* comes from the Latin word *inflamatio*, which means literally "to set on fire." The term is attributed to Aurus Cornelius Celsus, a Roman physician, who described the four characteristics of infected tissues: pain, redness, swelling, and warmth. An easily understood example of inflammation is a streptococcal throat infection (strep throat). In strep throat, a bacterial infection causes the throat to be red (inflamed) and sore, and may cause the throat to produce a whitish discharge (pus). Similarly, the colon or small intestine in Crohn disease or ulcerative colitis may be red and sore, with mucus and a white discharge (called *exudate*). Looking at inflamed tissue under the microscope, the physician sees many white blood cells.

In bacterial infections, such white blood cells are helpful in clearing the infection, but at times inflammation can be harmful. Harmful inflammation occurs when the body's immune system attacks the body's own tissues; any condition that causes this process is called an *autoimmune,* or *autoinflammatory,* disease. Examples of such illnesses include diabetes (where the immune system attacks the pancreas), psoriasis (where the immune system attacks the skin), and inflammatory bowel disease (where the immune system attacks the intestine). In ulcerative colitis, the pain, redness, and swelling are limited to the large intestine (colon). In Crohn disease, the inflammation can occur not only in the colon, but also in the small intestine and other areas of the gastrointestinal tract.

What Is Ulcerative Colitis?

Ulcerative colitis (UC) is a type of inflammatory bowel disease in which inflammation is usually found only in the large intestine. The term *ulcerative* is used because the patient has small breaks, called ulcers, in the lining of the colon when the disease is active, which causes the person to have symptoms. Ulcers are areas where the lining of the intestine has been so damaged that it has been worn away, leaving a small hole or sore. Shallow ulcers commonly occur in the large intestine in active ulcerative colitis. *Colitis* means inflammation (-itis) of the large intestine (colon). In children, ulcerative colitis usually involves the whole colon (*pancolitis*). In some children, however, the colitis affects only the left side of the large intestine (left-sided colitis), or the rectum (*ulcerative proctitis*). (See figure 1.4.)

The symptoms of ulcerative colitis—such as diarrhea, rectal bleeding, and abdominal pain—result directly from inflammation of the large intestine. The symptoms of ulcerative colitis vary over time. When a patient is having cramps, diarrhea, and rectal bleeding, she is usually having a "flare," an "exacerbation," or a period of "active disease." In contrast, when a patient feels well and has no significant digestive symptoms, the doctor will consider her to be in *remission*. In addition to gut symptoms, patients with IBD may also develop inflammation outside their GI tract, including joint swelling (*arthritis*), eye redness (*uveitis*), and skin rashes. Complications of IBD that occur in organs other than the intestine are called *extraintestinal symptoms*. These symptoms are discussed in more detail in chapter 12.

While ulcerative colitis is a lifelong illness, it can usually be well controlled with medications. During flareups (periods of disease activity), stronger medications may be needed. During periods of remission (inactive disease), milder medications (*maintenance therapies*) are often used. The course of the illness is also variable; some patients have more frequent flareups than other patients. In a small number of people, the disease does not respond well to medications, and surgical options may need to be considered (see chapter 11).

In summary, ulcerative colitis is a disease characterized by a typical pattern of inflammation in the large intestine. The most common symptoms during a flare are abdominal cramping, diarrhea, and rectal bleeding. The physician and the parent share the same goal: to control the child's illness in order to keep flares as short as possible and remissions as long as possible.

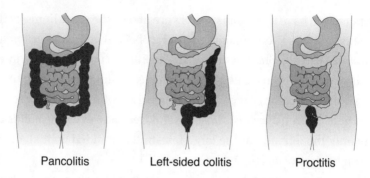

Pancolitis   Left-sided colitis   Proctitis

Common locations for ulcerative colitis

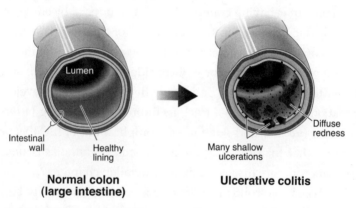

Normal colon
(large intestine)   Ulcerative colitis

Figure 1.4. Common locations for ulcerative colitis. The inflammation in ulcerative colitis is usually limited to the large intestine (colon). In most children, the entire colon is inflamed (pancolitis; *top left*). In about 25% of children, only the left side of the colon is affected (left-sided colitis, *middle*). In less than 10% of children, the inflammation is limited to the rectum (proctitis; *top right*). The inflammation in ulcerative colitis is characterized by a change in the normal colon's healthy lining (*bottom left*), making that inner lining red and ulcerated (*bottom right*).

What Is Crohn Disease?

Crohn disease (CD) is similar to ulcerative colitis, in that it causes inflammation of the intestines. The main difference between CD and UC is in the area of intestine most commonly involved. The disease in UC is limited to the large intestine. In contrast, CD can occur in any part of the GI tract, between the mouth and the anus. The most common places are the last portion of the small intestine (the terminal ileum) and the first part of the large intestine (the cecum). (See figure 1.5.)

A second major difference between Crohn disease and ulcerative colitis is that the inflammation in Crohn disease is often deeper, and involves the whole wall of the colon (*transmural inflammation*). The severity of the inflammation can vary from tiny ulcers to large, deep, and destructive ulcers. Most of the time, the ulcers are small and heal easily with medication. Sometimes, though, a deep ulcer forms a hole in the intestine, which leads to an abdominal infection, called an *abscess* (see figure 1.5). The abdominal abscess occurs because a hole in the intestine allows intestinal fluid to leak into the abdomen. Inflammation in Crohn disease can also cause an area of the bowel to be narrowed, or *strictured*, which can cause cramps and vomiting.

As with ulcerative colitis, Crohn disease is characterized by active periods (flares) and quiet periods (remission). However, the symptoms of CD may differ from the symptoms of UC. Because Crohn sometimes involves the small intestine but not the large intestine, patients with Crohn often have belly pain, fatigue, and weight loss without rectal bleeding. As with ulcerative colitis, the primary treatment for Crohn disease is medication, and the common aim of the physician and parent is to keep flares as short as possible and remission as long as possible. In addition to medication, some people may benefit from dietary therapy (see chapter 13), while others may benefit from surgery to remove a portion of the diseased intestine (chapter 11).

Indeterminate Colitis

At times, after a gastroenterologist has thoroughly tested a patient, the physician cannot tell whether the IBD is Crohn disease or ulcerative colitis. This usually occurs when the person has IBD that involves the large intestine (like UC) but has some features that suggest CD. These patients may be given a diagnosis of *indeterminate colitis* (IC, also

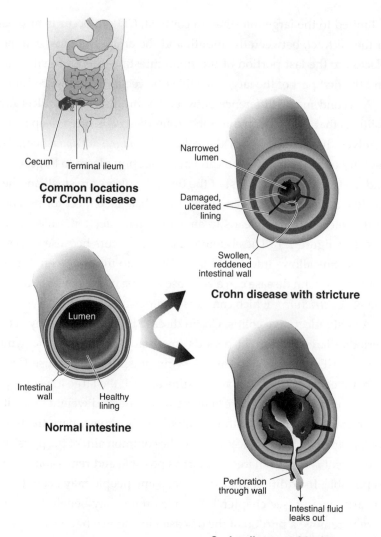

Cecum   Terminal ileum

**Common locations
for Crohn disease**

Narrowed
lumen

Damaged,
ulcerated
lining

Swollen,
reddened
intestinal wall

Crohn disease with stricture

Lumen

Intestinal
wall
Healthy
lining

Normal intestine

Perforation
through wall

Intestinal fluid
leaks out

Crohn disease with abscess

Figure 1.5. Crohn disease can involve any region of the intestine, but the most common area is the last part of the small intestine (the terminal ileum) and first part of the large intestine (the cecum). Over time, the inflammation may result in different complications. Some patients may develop a thick intestinal wall and a narrow lumen (stricture, *top right*), which results in an inability to pass food through the intestine (obstruction). Other patients with Crohn may develop a hole in the intestinal wall (perforation), resulting in leakage of intestinal fluid into the abdomen (abdominal abscess, *bottom right*).

called *IBD unclassified*). Often patients with IC are treated very much like patients with ulcerative colitis, then reevaluated later to see if their disease can now be called either Crohn or ulcerative colitis.

IBD may be subdivided into three main groups: ulcerative colitis, Crohn disease, and indeterminate colitis. Once diagnosed, most people with IBD can be treated with medications to get the disease under control (see chapter 10). Most children respond well to treatment and can lead a normal life. However, all children with IBD need long-term follow-up with a gastroenterology team for medical treatment, nutritional assessments, and emotional support.

❧ 2

IBD Causes and Risk Factors

IBD has been a topic of study by doctors and scientists for more than fifty years, but we still do not know precisely why people with IBD develop inflamed intestines. Scientists believe that both genetics and environment play major roles in the development of the disease. The interaction between genes and environment most likely activates (turns on) the cells of the immune system, causing the intestinal symptoms. This chapter will summarize what we know and what we don't know about causes of IBD. We are optimistic that future research will help us pinpoint the causes of these mysterious illnesses.

The Epidemiology of IBD

The term *epidemiology* refers to the study of disease distribution and frequency. Epidemiologists are scientists who ask questions such as these:

> Who gets a disease?
> How common is the disease?
> Are there any factors that put a person at risk for getting the
>   disease?

Epidemiologists have concluded, for example, that smokers have a greater risk of lung cancer than nonsmokers, and that African Americans are at higher risk for developing sickle cell disease than are Caucasians. Epidemiologists studying IBD have found an increased prevalence of the disease in certain races and ethnic groups. For example,

IBD is more common in Caucasians than in African Americans and Asians, and is also more common in people of Eastern European Jewish background. However, any person can develop IBD, regardless of their racial or ethnic background. Another observation epidemiologists have made about IBD is that it seems to be more common in countries farther away from the equator (northern latitudes) and less common in countries closer to the equator.

Epidemiologists estimate that over one million Americans have IBD. Thus, IBD affects 1 in every 300 Americans. Approximately 100,000 of those Americans with IBD are children. Studies from both the United States and other countries suggest that more and more people are being diagnosed with either Crohn disease or ulcerative colitis. One study in Finland found that the number of children with CD and UC had doubled in the last twenty years. Even in countries like India, where IBD was once unheard of, many people are being diagnosed with the condition. Therefore, IBD is no longer a rare disease, and there is evidence that it is becoming more common.

Family History and Genetics

It has been recognized for a long time that IBD seems to run in families. About 15 to 20 percent of people with IBD have close relatives with the disease. Evidence also suggests that people with IBD who develop their illness during childhood are more likely to have other family members with IBD, compared with people whose illness begins when they are adults. A very large study of adults with IBD living in Denmark found that the children of adults with IBD had a two to thirteen times higher risk of either Crohn disease or ulcerative colitis than did the children of parents without IBD. In addition, people with IBD may be more likely to have family members with other autoimmune diseases, such as thyroid disease or rheumatoid arthritis.

Nonetheless, IBD is not exclusively hereditary. We know that this is true from information gathered in identical twin studies. Among identical twins, when one twin develops Crohn disease, the likelihood of the other twin developing the same illness is about 50 percent. By contrast, if one identical twin develops ulcerative colitis, the other twin will develop UC only about 15 percent of the time. Therefore, although having an identical twin with IBD greatly increases a person's risk of developing IBD, in many twin pairs, one twin has IBD and the other doesn't.

Once it was understood that family history increases the risk of developing either CD or UC, formal genetic studies were done on families to gather more information. Geneticists are scientists who study how parental traits, or characteristics, are transmitted via genes to children. A mother and a father both transmit genes to their children, and every child is a combination of genes from both the mother and the father. The genetic material within cells that determines what characteristics a child will develop is called *deoxyribonucleic acid,* or DNA. A person's DNA acquired from mother and father will determine his height, eye color, and sex. Genes can also transmit risk of disease, which is how some diseases may run in families. In the case of Crohn disease and ulcerative colitis, there is no one gene or DNA piece that determines whether a child will develop these diseases. IBD is a *polygenic* disease; in other words, many genes (some from each parent) probably play a role.

IBD is also called a complex disease, which means both that there are many different types of IBD and that genes and environment together play a role in determining whether a person will get the disease. Environmental factors may determine if the disease will occur, when it will occur, and the types of signs and symptoms a person will show. Because IBD is a complex disease, identifying the specific genes that cause it is very difficult. In the past ten years, however, major progress has been made in studies of the heredity of IBD. In 2001, it was determined that about 25 percent of people with Crohn disease have an abnormal gene called NOD2 (otherwise known as CARD 15). More recent studies, involving large collaborations between many universities, have shown that over 30 genes may be associated with either Crohn disease or ulcerative colitis.

What precisely do these genes do? Although the function of the genes involved in IBD has yet to be resolved, current evidence suggests that these genes have at least two major functions:

1. The genes determine how the immune system cells react to intestinal bacteria. Bacteria are normally present in the intestine, but if the body's immune system sees these bacteria as invaders, or pathogens, inappropriate inflammation may occur.
2. The genes also determine how different cells of the immune system talk to each other (this is called *immune regulation*). Immune cells communicate with each other by chemicals called *cytokines*, or *chemokines*. If the wrong communication is going on between cells, inappropriate inflammation may occur.

There is no doubt that the genetics of IBD are very complex. The complexity of the genetics makes it unlikely that a genetic test for Crohn disease or ulcerative colitis will be developed in the near future. Still, unraveling the genetics may help us better understand what causes these conditions and how best to treat them.

The Environment

The studies of genetics in IBD are challenging, but research on environmental risk factors is even more challenging. Because IBD is a rare disease, scientists need to study large numbers of people to identify environmental risk factors. In addition, an environmental risk factor may not cause (or trigger) a disease until after many years *of* exposure (or until many years *after* an exposure). For example, it can take thirty years of a poor diet, smoking, and lack of exercise before a person develops diabetes or heart disease. The lapse of time between exposure and disease can make it difficult to prove the association (or link) between the environmental trigger and the onset of disease. IBD is clearly more common in the modern era, but many factors of modern life might be associated with the rise in IBD, including changes in diet, decreased physical activity, altered environmental bacteria, and decreased childhood infections. The section below summarizes the environmental risk factors that may play a role. The research in this area is inconclusive, however, and the precise environmental causes remain a topic of active study.

Diet and IBD

One of the first questions that parents ask after their child has been diagnosed with IBD is "What should my child eat?" Unfortunately, this is a very difficult question for a physician to answer. Unlike food allergies or celiac disease (a bowel disease triggered by an immunologic reaction to wheat, rye, and barley), IBD is not caused by a specific food. Some people report that certain foods may make them worse, but these foods vary from person to person. A physician or nutritionist cannot prescribe a diet that will help everyone, because:

- IBD is different for different individuals.
- Available research cannot agree on the role of diet in the development of IBD.
- Good studies are difficult to perform and often require remembering details of eating habits going back several years before diagnosis.
- The patient may have altered her diet at the beginning of symptoms, before a diagnosis was confirmed.

Some studies have shown a connection between eating processed hydrogenated fats, such as margarine, and the start of CD and UC. In Japan, the rise in IBD has correlated with a shift to a more Westernized diet lower in fish oil and higher in animal fat. Other studies have suggested that refined sugars and processed carbohydrates are associated with an increased risk of IBD and that higher intake of fruits and vegetables reduces the risk of developing the disease. Much more research is needed. When a child is newly diagnosed with IBD, the first instinct of the parent may be to modify the child's diet. Indeed, some children with Crohn disease will benefit from receiving a special liquid diet, called the elemental diet, under a physician's supervision (see chapter 13). Unfortunately, aside from the elemental diet, there is

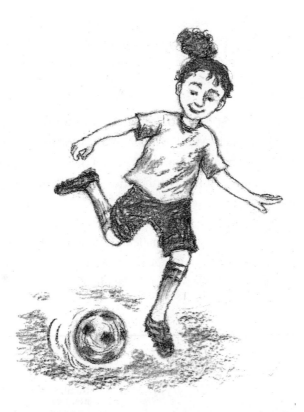

no conclusive medical evidence that modifying one's dietary intake *after* developing IBD will control the disease. Although many "special diets" that are supposed to treat IBD are available on the Internet and in the general press, these diets have not been well studied (chapter 21). These "alternative diets" may benefit some people, but they are not a substitute for conventional medical treatment.

Other Environmental Risk Factors

Many studies have shown that cigarette smoking is associated with a higher risk of developing Crohn disease and may be a risk factor for flares of Crohn disease. On the other hand, in ulcerative colitis, smoking may decrease the risk of flaring; the negative health effects of smoking far outweigh any effects smoking may have on UC flares, however, and it is strongly recommended that people with UC not smoke. Oral contraceptives may slightly increase the risk of Crohn disease in women, but most women with IBD can safely take oral contraceptives. Immunizations have not been associated with increased risk of developing IBD.

Intestinal Bacteria: An Overlooked "Environmental" Cause

Trillions of bacteria live in the lumen of the human intestine (figure 2.1); they populate the intestinal fluid but are kept out of the human body by the intestinal lining (epithelium). More than four hundred different species of bacteria can be found in the large intestine, and most of these bacteria are normal inhabitants (commensals) of the human body. They even have beneficial functions—they help us digest food and make certain vitamins (for example, vitamin K). These normal bacteria may help protect us against invasion by disease-

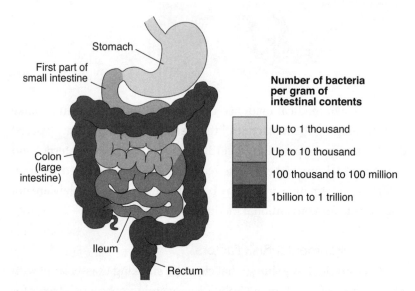

Figure 2.1. Bacteria living in the human intestine. The gastrointestinal tract is colonized by more than 100 trillion bacteria, and the numbers of bacteria increase farther down the intestine. The stomach and upper intestine have relatively few bacteria in the lumen, while the large intestine has trillions.

causing (pathogenic) bacteria. In most people, the "normal" bacteria populating the human intestine live peacefully in our bodies and do not cause inflammation.

What's different in people with IBD? Evidence is mounting that in people with IBD, the inflammation results when the person's immune system inappropriately responds to some of these normal bacteria. Some of the evidence comes from animal models. Mice that are genetically designed to develop colitis usually do not develop colitis when grown in germ-free, sterile environments. The colitis does not occur until the intestines of these mice are colonized with "normal" bacteria. In humans, antibiotics or other antibacterial treatments may reduce the severity of IBD, possibly by reducing the number of normal bacteria in the intestines. Many studies using sophisticated DNA fingerprinting technology are currently under way to determine whether some species of normal bacteria can cause IBD in humans.

Although bacteria may play a role in triggering IBD flares, many studies have failed to conclusively demonstrate a specific bacterial or viral "cause" of IBD. Organisms that have been studied include the tuberculosis bacteria, the nontuberculous atypical mycobacteria, clostridial species, and the measles virus. Almost all these studies have been inconclusive, and most scientists believe that IBD is not caused by one species of bacteria.

Increasing Cleanliness: The Hygiene Hypothesis

IBD, like a number of other immune-related diseases, may be the result of our society's improving cleanliness (the theory involving increasing cleanliness is called the *hygiene hypothesis*). In essence, over the past two to three decades, we have developed a wide range of products that take microbes away from our living space, from antibacterial soaps for washing dishes and laundry to antibiotics in our food sources. Thus, adults and children in countries with increasingly sterile environments are becoming more protected from routine infections (including chicken pox and *Salmonella*). Obviously, having protection from infections like chicken pox and *Salmonella* has many benefits;

these infections can make people very ill, and can even kill some of the people they infect.

But living in an overly clean environment might have drawbacks. Exposure to normal community-acquired infections may be important for the proper development of the immune system. The hygiene hypothesis proposes that lack of regular childhood infectious exposures might have a detrimental effect on the immune system, thus increasing the risk of immune-mediated diseases like diabetes, asthma, and IBD. Following this line of thought, some scientists hypothesize that overprotection from childhood infections may lead to the wrong immune response later in life. Although this hypothesis has not been proven, the combination of better living standards, lack of exposure to gut parasites, and exposure to new environmental factors could lead to increased vulnerability to IBD. In support of this theory, we find that people growing up on farms and exposed to farm animals in early childhood may be at lower risk for developing IBD.

Does Stress Cause IBD?

Stress is not the cause of IBD, but it may make symptoms worse. Some data show that chemicals (called *neuropeptides*) released by the brain and gut during periods of stress may increase the activity of the immune system. In addition, stressful situations may make a person less likely to go to the doctor or take his medications, which can result in flares of IBD. Managing stress and anxiety may therefore be helpful in controlling IBD symptoms.

The Immune System: IBD's Pathway

Whatever causes IBD, whether one factor or many, the result is that the body's own immune system inappropriately reacts against portions of the human intestine, causing inflammation. In the intestine of a person who has CD or UC, there are too many immune system cells. These cells damage normal gut tissues, resulting in redness, swelling, and ulcers of the intestinal lining, and causing the person to feel pain. Explaining all facets of how the immune system works requires a college semester and is beyond the scope of this book. For those interested, however, the section below will provide a brief summary of what the immune system is and how it "goes wrong" in IBD. This understanding may be helpful later in the book because most of our currently effective treatments for IBD work by reducing the activity of the immune system.

The intestine's immune system is designed mostly to repel harmful invaders (bacteria and viruses) from the body. Such invaders (for example, *Salmonella* and *E. coli* bacteria) are very common, yet relatively few people get sick from them, because the immune system is able to repel and kill the harmful bacteria. The major components of the immune system are the white blood cells that live in the blood, tissues, and intestinal lining. In the intestine, some white blood cells are free floating and others are clustered in *lymphoid nodules*. The cells of the immune system have different functions. Some cells are "lookouts" who sense invaders and notify the rest of the body: these include epithelial cells and dendritic cells. Other cells are "soldiers" who can move in and kill bacteria and viruses by eating them or by making antibodies. The main soldiers are called B cells, killer T cells, and macrophages. The last group of cells are the "master control cells"; they know when to turn the immune response on and off. Master control cells, like helper T cells, turn on the immune system when there is an infection, while other cells, called suppressor and regulatory T cells, turn off the immune system after the infection is over (figure 2.2).

Many different studies have examined what goes wrong in IBD to cause the patient's immune system to react against her intestine. As with other studies of what causes IBD, there is no single answer. In some people, the intestinal lookouts may react improperly to intestinal bacteria. In other cases, excessive antibodies may be made by soldier cells. In other cases, the master control cells may be altered, and once the immune system is turned on, it may be difficult (or impossible) to

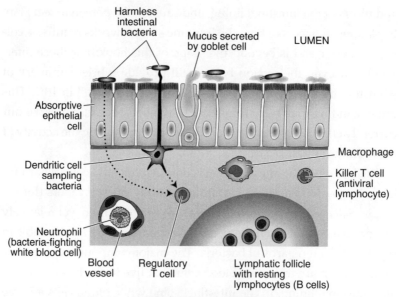

**Healthy intestinal lining
(magnified view)**

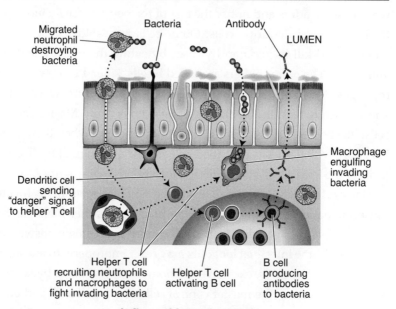

**Inflamed intestinal lining
(magnified view)**

turn off, resulting in uncontrolled inflammation. Knowledge gained by studying the genetics of IBD should ultimately help scientists who study the immune system answer many of these questions.

Scientists have made tremendous progress in understanding how intestinal inflammation comes about in IBD. However, there is still much more work to be done. Questions that have yet to be answered include the following:

1. Does any one gene or group of genes correlate with a specific type of IBD?
2. Which bacterial species, or groups of bacteria, might cause a genetically susceptible person to develop IBD?
3. Can bacterial populations in the intestine be altered through diet to decrease the risk of IBD?
4. Is there a way to reduce the activity of the immune system and control IBD without using medications that suppress the immune system?

These questions can be answered only through additional research. By participating in or funding research, parents can help doctors and scientists find the cause of IBD. We hope finding the cause may help prevent this disease in future generations.

Figure 2.2. *(opposite)* The lining of the intestine consists of cells that absorb nutrients (epithelial cells) and cells that produce intestinal mucus. Normally, bacteria are present both in the lumen and on the intestinal lining. Beneath the intestinal cell lining, there are normally several cells of the immune system that protect the body from infections (*top*). When the intestine is inflamed (*bottom*), more inflammatory cells (T cells, B cells, neutrophils) enter the intestinal wall.

3

Why Is It So Difficult to Diagnose IBD?

If your child has already been diagnosed with either Crohn disease or ulcerative colitis, her doctor will have already completed most of the health evaluation steps discussed in this chapter. Why, then, are we reviewing how doctors diagnose IBD? Because you may be wondering about the tests that have been done up to now and what they mean. Or you may have questions about how your doctor interprets these tests. Finally, you may be wondering, "Is the doctor right? Does my child really have IBD?"

This chapter reviews how health care professionals evaluate a child they suspect has IBD, and what tests will prove or disprove the diagnosis. While reading this chapter, keep in mind that at diagnosis, a patient with IBD must have evidence of inflammation and must have no evidence of an infection that would cause the inflammation. Evidence of inflammation may be seen

- at the time of physical examination
- on laboratory testing of blood or stool
- on x-ray
- during an endoscopic examination

If a child has no evidence of inflammation on testing, the child probably does not have IBD.

Symptoms and Signs That Make a Physician Suspect IBD

Ulcerative colitis and Crohn disease are different diseases that can affect different portions of the intestine. Significant inflammation in ulcerative colitis is usually seen only in the lower (large) intestine (colon). In contrast, Crohn disease can affect the large and small intestine. The vast majority of patients with ulcerative colitis (and indeterminate colitis) have the symptom of bloody diarrhea. In contrast, patients with Crohn disease often have less specific symptoms, including nonbloody diarrhea, weight loss, anemia, and tiredness.

IBD can be a sneaky disease, and for some people with IBD, a period of several months passes between the time symptoms start and the time of diagnosis. There are many reasons IBD can be sneaky, with a lag time to diagnosis. Symptoms may be mild and intermittent, for example. Also, many conditions far more common than IBD cause a symptom like belly pain. IBD may not come to the doctor's mind as a possibility when a person visits the doctor because of recurrent stomachaches. Before physicians can take steps to establish the diagnosis of IBD, they must first suspect that the person may have IBD.

IBD can be difficult to diagnose also because some children and teenagers who are embarrassed by the symptoms fail to tell their parents or the doctor what is really going on. Parents may be concerned about the invasiveness of tests such as colonoscopy and choose to "wait and see" before moving forward with testing. Another factor is that in a child with IBD, physical examinations and lab work are sometimes normal. In addition, some children with IBD may first see a doctor with symptoms outside the intestine—symptoms such as joint swelling, skin rashes, or eye inflammation.

Sometimes, though, IBD is anything but sneaky. Instead, it is extremely dramatic—for example, the child suddenly has severe bloody diarrhea as a symptom of ulcerative colitis. Bloody diarrhea is usually an alarming symptom that can frighten the child and the parent. Under these circumstances, a parent or child might ask for medical attention earlier rather than later. The doctor may need to rule out infection in the intestines before starting specific tests for IBD. (Some patients have both IBD and infection when their disease first causes symptoms.)

If the child's abdominal pain is mild and his general lifestyle and activity level are not affected, the correct diagnosis will often be delayed. Over time, as symptoms progress, it becomes easier to make the decision to start extensive testing. Table 3.1 lists some common symptoms and signs of IBD that are also seen in other diseases.

Table 3.1. Symptoms of IBD and other conditions

IBD symptom	What else might cause these symptoms?*
Anorexia (no appetite, refusing to eat)	• Anorexia nervosa
Weight loss, fatigue, or inability to keep up with peers	• Anemia • Malignancy (cancer) • Tuberculosis (TB)
Growth failure (not growing at a normal rate for the age) in a child with no other symptoms	• Endocrine (hormone) problems • Celiac disease
Repeated abdominal pain (stomachaches)	• Lactose intolerance • Infection with *Giardia* (a parasite) • Constipation • Functional abdominal pain
Persistent diarrhea	• Lactose intolerance • Infection with *Giardia* • Celiac disease
Bloody diarrhea	• Infections
Rectal bleeding	• Infections • Polyps (small growths in the colon)
Pain around the anus, with or without discharge	• Constipation • Hemorrhoids
Constipation	• Irritable bowel syndrome (IBS)
Joint pain or swelling	• Rheumatoid arthritis • Connective tissue diseases
Skin rash	• Infection • Connective tissue disease
Red eye	• Infection

* This list of other possible causes of these symptoms is not exhaustive. Other conditions can cause these symptoms, too.

Table 3.2. Tests used in diagnosing IBD

Name of Test	Type of Test	Purpose
Hematocrit	Blood	Measures blood count, looks for anemia
Erythrocyte sedimentation rate (esr)	Blood	Measures inflammation
C-reactive protein	Blood	Measures inflammation
Serologies (ANCA, ASCA)	Blood	Looks for antibodies some times seen in IBD patients
Stool culture	Stool	Looks for bacteria that can cause infectious colitis or sometimes trigger IBD
C. difficile toxin	Stool	Measures protein produced by C. difficile, a bacteria that can trigger IBD flares
Upper GI and small bowel series	Radiology	Uses x-rays to evaluate the small intestine for Crohn disease
Abdominal CT scan	Radiology	Uses x-rays to picture the intestines and the rest of the abdomen for IBD and infection
Abdominal MRI scan	Radiology	Uses magnetic imagery to picture the intestines and the rest of the abdomen for IBD and infection
Upper endoscopy	Scope	Uses a flexible tube inserted past the mouth and into the stomach to look for inflammation
Colonoscopy	Scope	Uses a flexible tube inserted past the anus and into the large intestine to look for inflammation
Biopsy	Microscope	Uses small tissue samples taken during endoscopy and colonoscopy to look for microscopic signs of Crohn disease or ulcerative colitis
Video capsule study	Capsule	Looks for difficult-to-find Crohn disease in the small intestine through a small "pill camera" that the patient swallows and that travels down the intestine, taking hundreds of pictures

Tests

A physician will suspect that a person may have IBD based on a combination of signs and symptoms. The most important initial evaluation is a thorough medical history and examination by a health care provider. The history and physical exam are described in chapter 6.

If the history and examination suggest either Crohn disease or ulcerative colitis, additional tests will need to be performed. These tests are important for several reasons:

- to confirm the diagnosis of IBD
- to exclude other conditions that might cause similar symptoms
- to differentiate between Crohn disease and ulcerative colitis
- to determine the severity of disease, which in turn guides treatment
- to evaluate other organ systems sometimes affected by inflammation, including the liver, skin, and eyes

Tests for IBD include blood tests, stool examinations, and x-rays. The definitive diagnosis of IBD is usually made by directly examining the stomach and upper part of the intestine with an endoscope (in a test called an *upper endoscopy*), and by examining the colon and ileum with a colonoscope (*colonoscopy*). During these tests, small samples from the intestine can be obtained for a pathologist to examine under a microscope. (Tissue taken during tests such as these is called a *biopsy*.) In patients for whom the diagnosis is strongly suspected but other tests are normal, a specialized device called a *video capsule*, or *pill camera*, may be used to take pictures of the small intestine. Table 3.2 summarizes the common tests physicians order when diagnosing and following complications of IBD. These tests are discussed in detail in Part II.

Part II
Diagnosing IBD

4

The Symptoms of IBD

After a child is diagnosed, two of the most common concerns a parent has are "How do I know when my child is sick?" and "How do I know what to worry about?" Because children and teens with IBD can develop other gastrointestinal illnesses, parents and physicians may also have trouble distinguishing between another type of illness and a flare. This chapter reviews some of the common symptoms seen in children and the various causes of these symptoms. As a general guideline, if an abdominal symptom is similar to what the child had when she first became ill, it's very often a flare of the disease. If an abdominal symptom is different in location, severity, duration, or nature, then it might be a new condition.

Abdominal Pain

Pain in the abdomen (stomach or belly area) is a common first symptom of IBD in 80 percent of people. But complaints of abdominal pain in children are very common, and children with IBD can have abdominal pain for many reasons. Abdominal pain can be minor and not important, or it can be a sign of a serious problem.

Abdominal pain can result from a variety of conditions affecting various organs. The characteristics of the pain—where it hurts, when it starts, how long it lasts, and how severe it is—are all important in helping to diagnose the cause. Any long-lasting or severe abdominal pain should be evaluated by a doctor. Table 4.1 lists causes of abdominal pain in children with ulcerative colitis and Crohn disease. Some of

Table 4.1. Some causes of abdominal pain in children with IBD

IBD Related

- Inflammatory pain (both Crohn disease and ulcerative colitis)
- Abdominal abscess (Crohn disease only)
- Bowel obstruction (usually in Crohn disease or after surgery)

IBD Unrelated, Serious	*IBD Unrelated, Usually Less Serious*
• Gallstones	• Constipation
• Pancreatitis	• Recurrent abdominal pain of
• Appendicitis	childhood (RAP)
• Kidney stones	• Irritable bowel syndrome (IBS)
• Gynecological problems	• Muscle or bone pain
• Peptic (stomach) ulcers	• Gastroesophageal reflux (GER)
	• Lactose intolerance

these problems are complications of the IBD itself, while others occur in children without IBD as well as in children with IBD.

Causes of Abdominal Pain Related to the Underlying IBD

Inflammatory Pain

Inflammatory pain occurs when a region of small intestine or colon remains swollen, red, and sore. This type of pain can be seen in either Crohn disease or ulcerative colitis. When the inflammation involves the colon (as in UC), pain typically occurs around the time of bowel movements and is accompanied by diarrhea or blood. In Crohn disease limited to the small intestine, however, the child does not necessarily have pain and diarrhea with the inflammation. Inflammatory pain is a sign of a "flare," or a sign that the IBD may need to be treated more aggressively. Figure 4.1 shows areas of the abdomen that may become inflamed: the colon, ileum, kidney, liver, gallbladder, or pancreas.

Abdominal Abscess

An abdominal abscess (intra-abdominal infection) is a complication of Crohn disease; children with ulcerative colitis almost never get one. An abdominal abscess is formed when Crohn disease causes a

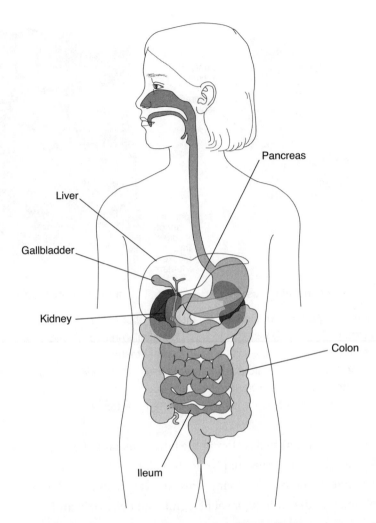

Figure 4.1. Digestive system with areas of abdomen that may become in-flamed. Abdominal pain can result from inflammation of many different organs, not just the intestine. Physicians can often guess what the problem is based on the location of the pain. For example, the pancreas is located in the upper abdomen, the gallbladder is located in the right upper abdomen, and the kidneys are located in the flank.

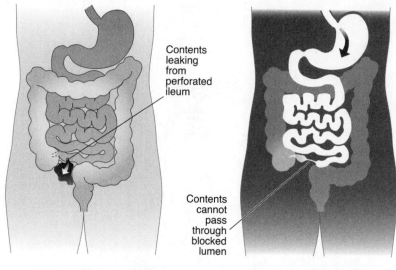

Abdominal abscess **Intestinal obstruction**

Figure 4.2. Abdominal abscess and intestinal obstruction. These two complications of Crohn disease usually result from inflammation in the small intestine. In an abdominal abscess, a hole in the intestine (usually the ileum) results in the leakage of fluid into the abdomen, mimicking what is seen in a
perforated appendix. In an intestinal obstruction (stricture), an area of the
intestine becomes scarred, so that contents have trouble passing.

hole (perforation) to develop in the bowel, usually the small intestine
(figure 4.2). When intestinal contents leak through the perforation, an
infection develops. The symptoms are very similar to appendicitis
and include the sudden onset of significant belly pain and fever.

Bowel Obstruction

A bowel obstruction means that food and fluid are having trouble
moving through the bowel because of a mechanical blockage. In CD
(but not in UC), obstructions may develop if the small intestine scars
internally and becomes narrow. Another cause of a bowel obstruction
is adhesions (kinks in the bowel that may occur after surgery). Children with obstructions typically have a sudden onset of belly pain and
vomiting, and the symptoms should be treated as an emergency. A

careful physical examination and abdominal x-ray will make it possible to diagnose most obstructions.

Serious Causes of Abdominal Pain Unrelated to IBD

Gallstones

Gallstones are seldom a cause of abdominal pain in children and teens. The gallbladder is a small sac located next to the liver that helps store digestive juices. Small stones can form inside the sac and irritate the gallbladder or tubes that drain the liver, causing pain. Gallstones can also cause inflammation of the pancreas (see pancreatitis, below) if the stone blocks the flow of digestive juices out of the pancreas. Gallbladder pain can be either sharp or dull and is usually felt on the right side of the abdomen, under the ribcage. Pain from the gallbladder usually starts a few minutes after a meal, especially if the meal is high in fat. Most gallstones can be easily detected by an ultrasound. If recurrent abdominal pain is the result of gallstones, the gallstones and gallbladder should be removed.

Pancreatitis

Pancreatitis is inflammation of a digestive organ called the pancreas, which is in the middle of the abdomen. The inflammation causes an injury to the pancreas. In children, pancreatitis may occur without explanation, but it can also be caused by gallstones, infections, and medications. Some of the medicines used to treat inflammatory bowel disease, such as azathioprine, 6-mercaptopurine, and 5-aminosalicylates, can cause pancreatitis. Children with Crohn disease can also develop pancreatitis due to inflammation of their small intestine.

Children with pancreatitis typically have a sudden onset of abdominal pain, back pain, or vomiting. People with IBD say that the pain from pancreatitis is "different" from the pain of a flare. The diagnosis of pancreatitis can usually be easily established with a blood test; an ultrasound or CT scan is often done to exclude gallstones. Pancreatitis usually goes away after a few hours or days of intravenous fluids. If it is suspected that a medication is causing the pancreatitis, then the medication will probably need to be discontinued.

Appendicitis

Appendicitis is the most common condition requiring emergency abdominal surgery in children, but it can occur at any age. Appendicitis happens when the inside of the appendix is blocked, leading to reduced blood flow away from the area. Classic symptoms of appendicitis include fever, nausea, vomiting, and pain. It can be difficult to distinguish appendicitis from a flare in children with Crohn disease, although appendicitis usually has a more sudden onset than a flare. Tests such as ultrasound and CT scans are helpful. The treatment of acute appendicitis is surgery to remove the appendix. Surgery usually happens within several hours after confirming the diagnosis.

Kidney Stones

Kidney stones can occur in anyone, but they are more common in people with Crohn disease. The symptoms of kidney stones include back and side pain, vomiting, and blood in the urine. The stones usually can easily be seen with an ultrasound. The standard treatment is intravenous fluid and pain medication.

Gynecological Problems

Gynecological problems (problems involving the female reproductive organs) can cause abdominal pain in teenage girls. These problems include pelvic infections or inflammation, sexually transmitted diseases, abnormal periods, pregnancy, or diseases of the ovaries. The pain can be located in the middle of the abdomen, or only in the lower right or left side; if the pain is in the lower abdomen, it may resemble IBD pain. Cysts on the ovaries can cause lower abdominal pain halfway through a girl's cycle. Tests for gynecological problems include urinalysis (checking the urine), urine culture, pregnancy testing, and a pelvic exam and screening for infections.

Peptic (Stomach and Duodenal) Ulcers

Ulcers are wounds that can occur in the stomach or lining of the intestine. In healthy people, they most commonly occur in the stomach or the first part of the small intestine. Ulcers occur in people with Crohn disease and in people with ulcerative colitis, though they occur more often in people with Crohn disease. If a person with IBD has been taking aspirin or steroids for a long time, then medication may be the cause of the peptic ulcer. The most common symptoms of an ulcer are pain and bleeding.

Less Serious Causes of Pain Unrelated to IBD

Constipation

Constipation is one of the most common reasons that children visit the pediatrician's office because of abdominal pain. While IBD most often causes diarrhea, some patients with IBD may also have constipation. Constipation can sometimes cause severe pain—it can feel like, or be mistaken for, appendicitis. Constipation can be diagnosed by taking a careful history, by performing a physical examination (including sometimes a rectal exam), and by checking an abdominal x-ray. Treatment of constipation in children usually involves giving them stool softeners and increasing the amount of fluid and fiber in their diet.

Recurrent Abdominal Pain

Recurrent abdominal pain (RAP) of childhood is a condition in which a child has repeated bouts of abdominal pain without an obvious physical explanation. By definition, children with RAP have at least three episodes of abdominal pain over at least three months. This definition applies to children who are three years or older. The pain is usually severe enough to get in the way of daily activities, but it does not have a clear cause. RAP affects nearly 11 percent of school-age children. More girls than boys are affected by RAP. The pain usually occurs only around the belly button area and is usually vague (not easy to localize); a short rest can be enough to relieve the pain. Treatment with antacids or pain relievers does not usually help. Doctors think that about 25 percent of children with RAP may grow up to have irritable bowel syndrome.

Irritable Bowel Syndrome

Irritable bowel syndrome (IBS) is one of the most common conditions affecting the bowel, affecting an estimated 15 percent of people in the United States. IBS is also known as spastic colon. Some doctors may call IBS "colitis" (inflammation of the large intestine), but the term is inaccurate here, because there is no inflammation. Symptoms of IBS include looser and more frequent bowel movements, straining while passing stool, urgency, and bloating. The pain often starts after eating. Distinguishing between IBS and IBD requires knowing all of the person's medical history, as well as using laboratory tests. If there is no anemia (low red blood cell count) and no signs of inflammation in special blood tests, the problem is probably IBS. In children who have IBD, however, colonoscopy may be needed to distinguish between an IBD flare and IBS.

Muscle or Bone Pain

Muscle or bone pain is not unusual after exercise. It can be difficult to tell the difference between exercise-related pain and more serious causes of abdominal pain. In exercise-related pain, there should be no trouble with bowel movements, no vomiting or fever, and the pain should get better after taking simple pain relievers such as acetaminophen or ibuprofen.

Gastroesophageal Reflux

Gastroesophageal reflux (GER) can cause abdominal pain, usually in the middle of the upper abdomen and spreading up into the chest. There may be nausea, or a feeling of food coming up into the esophagus (food pipe) and mouth. The pain often starts 30 minutes to 1 hour after a meal, especially a large meal, but it can occur at any time. Specific foods, such as carbonated drinks, caffeine, and tomato products, can make GER worse. Antacids can help decrease discomfort. Patients with IBD may also have symptoms of GER, especially if the IBD affects the stomach or esophagus.

Lactose Intolerance

Lactose intolerance can cause abdominal pain with increased intestinal gas and diarrhea. Lactose, or milk sugar, is found in dairy products and in most baked goods. About 20 percent of Caucasian adults, and up 80 percent of African American and Asian Americans, have lactose intolerance. People with IBD, particularly older children and young adults, may also have lactose intolerance. People who are lactose intolerant have trouble digesting the sugar in milk products. When they eat products containing milk, they develop symptoms of pain, gas, diarrhea, and bloating 30 to 60 minutes after meals. Treatment of lactose intolerance involves cutting back on milk products and taking pills that contain lactase enzyme (for example, Lact-Aid). Lactose intolerance is not an allergy to milk, and many lactose intolerant individuals can tolerate small to moderate amounts of milk or cheese.

Diarrhea

The previous section discussed different causes of abdominal pain and described the clues to help decide if the pain is caused by an IBD flare or another illness. Similarly, this segment will help describe the clues to help tell the difference between an IBD flare and another cause of diarrhea.

There are many different causes of diarrhea (table 4.2). Some of these conditions may feel like flares of Crohn disease and ulcerative colitis. If the cause of the diarrhea is unclear, your child's doctor can examine him and order laboratory tests. The physical exam and laboratory tests can usually determine the cause of the child's symptoms—whether it is IBD or something else.

Table 4.2. Causes of diarrhea in children with IBD

Bloody Diarrhea	Nonbloody Diarrhea

• Flareup of IBD
• Acute bacterial infections:
  Salmonella
  Shigella
  Campylobacter
  Yersinia
  E. coli
• C. difficile infection
• Amoeba infection (in people who recently traveled to areas of the world where this organism is common)
	• Irritable bowel syndrome
	• Lactose intolerance
	• Diarrhea after bowel surgery, due to rapid transit (food moving too fast through the intestines) too much bile acid in the colon malabsorption (inability of the small intestine to absorb important vitamins and other nutrients from food) bacterial overgrowth (too many bacteria in the intestines)
	• Prescribed medications
	• Herbs and dietary supplements
	• Too much juice or sugarless gum
	• Celiac disease
	• Excessive laxatives

Bloody Diarrhea

Bloody diarrhea with cramps is one of the most common symptoms of IBD. Very often, in a child who has been diagnosed with ulcerative colitis or Crohn disease colitis, the physician will simply treat for an IBD flare. Even so, it is important always to consider infection as a cause of the diarrhea, especially if the episode starts suddenly. A number of common bacterial infections can cause bloody diarrhea, including *Salmonella, Shigella, Campylobacter, Yersinia,* and *E. coli.* These infections usually occur when a person eats contaminated food. Especially risky are undercooked chicken (which can contain *Salmonella* and *Campylobacter*) and undercooked ground beef (which can contain *E. coli*).

Another bacterium that can cause bloody diarrhea is *Clostridium difficile* (*C. difficile,* often referred to as *C. diff*). This infection often occurs when a person has recently received antibiotics or has recently been hospitalized. C. difficile infection is common in people with IBD and can recur after treatment is stopped. When people travel abroad, bloody diarrhea (colitis) can also be caused by organisms not commonly seen in the United States, such as amoeba. Thus, it is important to inform your doctor if your family has traveled abroad recently.

Treatment is determined by which infection is causing the diarrhea. The cause of bacterial and amoebic colitis can usually be identified by a single stool culture, though multiple stool cultures may be necessary. A stool culture means checking to see if any organisms (for example, bacteria) grow in the stool. Special tests are needed to identify *C. difficile* and amoebic colitis. Unlike IBD colitis, most cases of bacterial colitis usually disappear on their own or get better with antibiotic treatment. In people with IBD, bleeding from the anus that lasts more than two weeks with negative cultures is probably due to an IBD flare.

Nonbloody diarrhea

Nonbloody diarrhea is very common in the general population and has many different causes. Most people with ulcerative colitis usually have bleeding in addition to diarrhea when their disease flares. On the other hand, people with Crohn disease (particularly Crohn disease in the small intestine) can have nonbloody diarrhea, especially if they have had bowel surgery.

Acute nonbloody diarrhea (a sudden attack of mushy or watery diarrhea) is usually caused by a virus. Viruses generally affect the lining of the small intestine, causing oozing of intestinal fluid. Viruses also limit the absorption (taking in) of food from the small intestine. Viral infections of the intestines often spread from person to person, mainly through saliva or infected stools. For example, viral infection of the intestines spreads rapidly among young children in daycare settings. A stool sample can easily identify some of these viruses but not others. Nausea, vomiting, and low-grade fevers (usually 101° or less) are normal in children with viral illnesses. Diarrhea from a viral infection usually lasts between three to seven days, though some illnesses can last as long as fourteen days.

In people without IBD, chronic nonbloody diarrhea is most commonly caused by either irritable bowel syndrome (IBS) or lactose intolerance (see previous section on abdominal pain unrelated to IBD).

The results of diagnostic tests, including blood tests, stool cultures, and colonoscopy (see chapters 7–9), are normal in people with IBS. These normal tests help distinguish IBS from the different forms of inflammatory bowel disease. To complicate things somewhat, however, patients with IBD (either Crohn disease or ulcerative colitis) can also have IBS. In some cases, the best way to tell the difference between symptoms arising from IBS and those from a mild flare of IBD is with a colonoscopy. If the colonoscopy and biopsies suggest that the IBD is under control, then IBS should be treated.

Chronic diarrhea can occur in patients who have had bowel surgery for Crohn disease. This is true especially when the last part of the small intestine (terminal ileum) and first part of the large intestine (cecum) were surgically removed. The diarrhea occurs in part because things move through the shorter intestine more quickly, and in part because bile acids (digestive chemicals in the intestine) may irritate the colon. In any person with Crohn disease who has had this surgery and develops chronic nonbloody diarrhea, the first step is to make sure that the disease is not flaring. If a flare is ruled out, then diarrhea after surgery can be treated with the medication cholestyramine (Questran) to reduce the bile acids. Additional helpful medications are loperamide (Imodium), to slow down the movement of food through the intestines, and metronidazole (Flagyl) if there are too many bacteria in the intestines.

When the intestines are not able to take in everything the body needs from the food the person eats, this is called *malabsorption*. Malabsorption can occur if there is widespread Crohn disease of the small intestine, or if major surgery was done on the small intestine. Malabsorption may require a modified diet and vitamin supplements.

Other causes of diarrhea do not commonly affect children with IBD. Some prescription medications for IBD, such as 5-ASA, may cause diarrhea. In addition, over-the-counter treatments such as herbal and dietary supplements may cause diarrhea. Too much juice and sugarless gum can result in a mushy or watery diarrhea. Celiac disease, a form of intolerance to wheat, can cause diarrhea, abdominal pain, and gas; the diagnosis can be established by a simple blood test and an upper endoscopy. Finally, some people with IBD may at times feel constipated; if they take too many laxatives, they may develop diarrhea.

Slowed Growth and Late Puberty

Many chronic inflammatory diseases can cause slowed growth and delayed puberty (growth failure). This is particularly true in children with IBD. Approximately 50 percent of children with Crohn disease

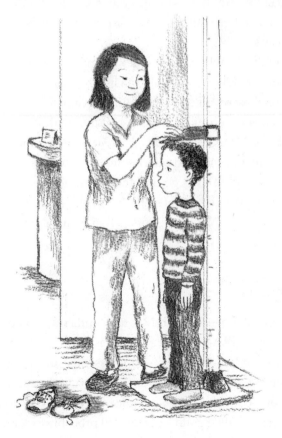

Measuring a child's height at each clinic visit is very important, especially for children with Crohn disease and growth failure.

Table 4.3. Causes of slow growth and late puberty in children with IBD

- Poor intake resulting in too few calories, caused by
  abdominal pain
  decreased appetite
  fear of eating
  nutrient deficiencies
- Inflammation's effects on puberty: direct suppression of puberty by
  inflammatory chemicals (cytokines)
- Poor absorption of food and calories, caused by
  loss of intestine from surgery
  decreased nutrient absorption because of intestinal inflammation
  specific vitamin deficiencies

and 10 percent of children with ulcerative colitis will develop such symptoms. Slowed growth and delayed puberty may be the first sign of Crohn disease.

A child with IBD who is smaller and skinnier than his classmates, or whose predicted height is smaller than what his parents would expect based on their own heights, should be evaluated for growth failure. The reasons for growth failure in children with IBD are summarized in table 4.3. Fundamentally, chronic inflammation suppresses appetite, leading to decreased calories, which in turn causes undernutrition. Because the child is getting fewer calories than desired, her growth slows. Prolonged use of steroids can also result in growth failure through a direct effect on the bones. Treatment of growth failure is discussed in chapter 13.

Liver Problems

About 5 percent of people with IBD have inflammation of the liver. The liver is a triangular-shaped organ that is located in the upper right portion of the abdomen. This organ is essential in digesting foods, making proteins, and ridding the body of toxins. Symptoms of liver disease include chronic fatigue, jaundice (a yellow color to the skin), and severe itching. Your child's doctor will probably order blood tests to check liver function at least once a year. The digestive juices made in the liver leave the liver and enter the intestine through a series of tubes called bile ducts (figure 4.3). Primary sclerosing cholangitis (PSC) is an inflammatory disorder of the bile ducts that can cause scarring and blockages within the ducts; it occurs more commonly in UC than in CD, but it can also occur in CD. For many patients, PSC is a mild condition that can be treated with medication. Over time, though, some patients with PSC develop liver cirrhosis (scarring of the liver).

Autoimmune hepatitis (AIH) is another liver disorder that some

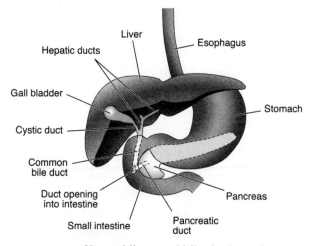

Normal liver and bile ducts

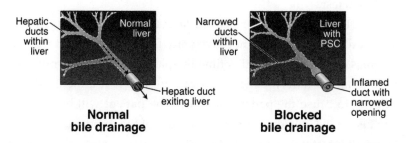

Figure 4.3. The liver produces digestive juices (bile) that enter a series of small tubes called hepatic ducts and bile ducts. The digestive juices then enter the upper part of the intestine (duodenum). In a rare condition called primary sclerosing cholangitis (PSC), which a few people with IBD develop, the ducts draining the liver become narrowed and scarred.

people with IBD develop. In AIH, the body's immune system attacks the liver cells, similar to the way it attacks the intestine in Crohn disease. Most people with Crohn disease and AIH have no symptoms of hepatitis, and although the liver tests your child has every year will also screen for AIH, only a liver biopsy can confirm the diagnosis of AIH. Drug treatment of autoimmune hepatitis with the medications prednisone and azathioprine usually controls the disease.

People with IBD, especially Crohn disease, are prone to develop gallstones (cholelithiasis). The risk increases if they are not allowed to take in food or drinks by mouth for a period, for example, if they get nutrition through a vein (known as *parenteral nutrition*), or if they require treatment with corticosteroids.

Pancreas Problems

Pancreatitis (inflammation of the pancreas) can develop in people with IBD for several reasons. The most common is a reaction to medications that are commonly used to treat IBD. Medications known to trigger pancreatitis include sulfasalazine, mesalamine, azathioprine, and 6-mercaptopurine. In pancreatitis, the inflamed pancreas causes severe abdominal pain and vomiting. The diagnosis is easily made by the identification of elevated pancreatic proteins (amylase and lipase) in a blood test.

A typical episode of pancreatitis lasts three to five days. To treat pancreatitis, the patient is not given any food by mouth, so that the pancreas can rest. During this time the patient will receive nutrition through an IV. Rarely, pancreatitis can be severe. If a medication is believed to cause the pancreatitis, then the patient will be asked to stop taking it. Gallstones or Crohn disease of the duodenum (part of the small intestine) can block the pancreatic duct, also causing pancreatitis. Because the pain of pancreatitis can feel like the pain of severe IBD, a careful physical and diagnostic examination is required when pancreatitis is suspected to determine the true source of the symptoms.

Symptoms from Organs Outside the Gastrointestinal Tract

Joint Pain and Inflammation

Joint pain (*arthralgia*) and joint inflammation (*arthritis*) are the most common IBD symptoms that occur outside the intestines. The knees, hips, and ankles are the joints most likely to suffer (figure 4.4). Joint pain and joint inflammation tend to come at the same time as inflammation in the intestines. In some cases, however, joint problems may show up before the diarrhea and abdominal pain connected with IBD. The joints may ache and be painful without any obvious change in how they look. When serious inflammation is present, the joint will appear swollen, warm to the touch, or red. There may also be pain when the joint is used or examined. Very often, joint disease improves

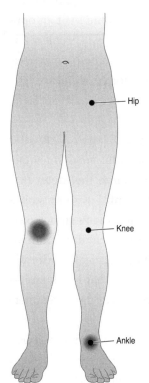

Figure 4.4. People with IBD may develop joint pain or swelling. Usually, large joints (hip, knee, ankle) are affected. In addition, the joint swelling is usually asymmetric (affecting one joint, but not the same joint on the opposite side).

when the IBD is controlled. When the joint inflammation does not respond to treatment of the IBD, the child may benefit from consulting a pediatric rheumatologist (arthritis specialist).

Eye Problems

The eye becomes inflamed in a small percentage of children with IBD. In *episcleritis*, the most common eye problem, the sclera (white of the eye) and the conjunctiva (the inside of the eyelid and the covering in front of the eyeball) become reddened and inflamed. There is no pain or change in eyesight. This condition may look like pink eye. In *uveitis*, inflammation of the uvea (the middle part of the eye) causes significant pain, and the vision can become blurry and sensitive to light.

Both conditions, and particularly uveitis, require treatment by an ophthalmologist (eye doctor). The seriousness of the eye problem is not always related to the seriousness of the IBD. While eye problems are uncommon in children with IBD, your child should visit an ophthalmologist (eye doctor) regularly to identify any eye problems as early as possible. Your child's gastroenterologist can help you determine how often eye exams should be scheduled for your child.

Kidney Problems

Kidney stones may develop in people with IBD, particularly after surgery that involves the ileum, the last section of the small intestine. The passage of a kidney stone from the kidney into the ureter (the tube that carries urine to the bladder) is very painful. Kidney stones are usually diagnosed with ultrasound. Although many stones pass normally during urination, after the person receives hydration treatment, kidney stones may need to be removed surgically. Alternatively, a technique called *lithotripsy* (sound waves that break stones into smaller pieces so that they can pass normally through the ureter) may be used.

Other, rarer kidney problems that may occur in CD (but not in UC) include blockage of the ureter by an inflammatory growth, and *fistulas* (abnormal openings) between the intestines and the bladder.

Skin Problems

People with IBD may develop skin rashes, some of which are associated with inflammation. *Erythema nodosum* is a rash of painful red bumps on the shins that appears in children with new onset or flaring IBD. A more severe rash, *pyoderma gangrenosum*, causes large ulcers but is very rarely seen in children. Some medications (for example, sulfasalazine) may increase sensitivity to sunlight, which makes the child more likely to get sunburned. Children with IBD may also develop allergic reactions to their medications, which look like "drug rashes."

Children with ulcerative colitis or Crohn disease can experience many different symptoms. In some children, warning signs of a flare are obvious. In others, warning signs may be subtle. In addition, some children may visit the doctor because they think they have a flare, only to be diagnosed with some other illness. Because this happens so often, it's not a good idea to assume that every GI symptom is a flare of IBD. Both patients and physicians need to consider other diagnoses, and additional testing should be performed if needed to make a diagnosis. It is crucial for children with UC who are having new diarrhea to have stool cultures performed to rule out infections.

✖ 5

How to Prepare for a Visit to Your Child's IBD Doctor

Caring for a child with IBD involves a partnership between the parent and the physician. The parent and the physician work together to keep the child's IBD under control. The parent's role is to provide accurate information, ask questions, gain knowledge, and provide input into decisions about the child's treatment. The physician's responsibility is to provide accurate information, ask questions, examine the patient, assess disease severity, and recommend a treatment plan. Physicians and parents need to discuss alternatives and make choices together.

Most children with IBD in North America are cared for by pediatric gastroenterologists. A pediatric gastroenterologist is a doctor who specializes in the diagnosis and management of diseases of the digestive system in people up to age 16, 18, or sometimes 21 years. A good resource to find a pediatric gastroenterologist is the Web site of the North American Society for Pediatric Gastroenterology, Hepatology, and Nutrition: www.naspghan.org. If you are reading this book, then most likely you have already consulted with a pediatric gastroenterologist. At what age a child stops seeing a pediatric gastroenterologist and starts seeing an adult gastroenterologist depends on the geographic location or institution in which the patient is being seen. Older children and teens may be cared for by a gastroenterologist who treats mostly adult patients.

Preparing for a First Visit to the Gastroenterologist

Seeing a new doctor for the first time can be exciting, especially if there's a possibility that the doctor will have new or helpful ideas to improve the child's health or well being. But this visit can also be an unsettling time for parents and children, especially if they are changing from one medical practice to another or have moved to a new city or town. Some families may be reading this book while in the process of changing from an adult to a pediatric gastroenterologist (or vice versa), changing from one pediatric gastroenterologist to another, or moving from one town to another. Many families are happy with their current care but want to obtain another opinion about medical treatment. Whether for a first visit to a new doctor or a return visit, a parent can do much to help make the most of each appointment, and to help the doctor, as well. Careful preparation is the key.

The parent who arrives prepared makes it much more likely that three important goals can be reached during that first critical visit with the doctor:

1. Your gastroenterologist (and gastroenterology nurse practitioner, where applicable) will have in hand all the important medical history and test results and therefore will be better prepared to determine how to manage your child's IBD.
2. Your child will know what to expect during the visit, which will help her cooperate with the medical team.
3. Your key concerns and questions will be addressed.

How can you and your child prepare for the doctor's visit so that you can achieve the three goals listed above? Gather a history of your child's illness, get copies of medical records, and write down your questions and concerns.

Step 1. Assemble a complete a history of your child's illness as well as relevant family illnesses. Try to make these histories as complete as possible.

    A. Review in your own mind your child's current illness and describe it in writing.
- When did it begin?
- How often do the symptoms occur?
- How has your child been functioning: energy level, appetite, school performance, sleep?
- Have you been aware of any fevers?
- Do you think your child has lost weight?

    B. Sit down with your child in a quiet place, away from distractions, and compare notes about when his problems and symptoms started, and how things are going now. Be prepared to discuss these topics with your child:
- Pain
  When does it happen?
  Where is it located?
  How severe is it?
  How long does it last?
  What brings it on or relieves it?
- Weight changes
- Energy level
- Sleep
- Appetite
- School performance (Has it changed due to physical discomfort?)
- Aching joints
- Fevers
- Mouth sores
- Bowel movements (stools). This is often the most difficult subject for your child to talk about:
  How many a day?

What do they look like? (including any visible blood or mucus)

Are they painful?

Do they occur at night?

Are there any sores around your child's bottom?

It can be very helpful to the physician for you to inspect your child's bowel movements a couple of times before the first visit.

C. Keep a diary of symptoms, including stools (detailed as above), for one to two weeks before the visit.

D. Make a list of all your child's medications and doses (bring this list to the doctor). Be sure to include vitamin supplements, herbal products, and any nutritional supplements your child is taking. (You can also bring all the pill containers to the doctor's office so that he or she can read the labels, if desired.)

E. Think about your child's medical history. Has your child ever been hospitalized, or had surgery? Is your child allergic to any medications or foods?

F. Contact your relatives—grandparents, aunts, uncles, first cousins of your child—and ask about a history of any of the following:

- Inflammatory bowel disease (Crohn disease, ulcerative colitis)
- Primary sclerosing cholangitis (a liver disease affecting the bile ducts, often causing yellowing of the skin and eyes)
- Irritable bowel syndrome (spastic colon)
- Lactose intolerance

Step 2. Obtain copies of essential medical records and test results.

A. General health information from the primary care doctor or nurse practitioner that will be helpful to the GI team includes
- childhood illnesses
- growth chart
- immunization records

B. Previous blood tests, which may include
- complete blood count (CBC)

- protein level (albumin)
- markers of inflammation—sedimentation rate, CRP (C-reactive protein)
- liver function tests (AST/SGOT, ALT/SGPT, bilirubin levels, alkaline phosphatase)

C. Stool tests, which may include
- stool culture
- *Clostridium difficile* (*C diff* toxin)
- ova and parasites (O & P)
- *Giardia*

D. X-rays, which may include
- plain abdominal films (acute abdominal series and kidneys, ureter, and bladder, also called KUB)
- upper gastrointestinal series (UGI) with small bowel series (also called UGI with small bowel follow through)
- abdominal CT (CAT) scan
- magnetic resonance imaging (MRI)

Bring copies of the actual films, if possible, as well as the radiologist's official report. Your primary care doctor will generally not have a copy of the actual films; you can get a copy from the laboratory or hospital where the x-rays were done.

E. Procedures, which may include
- upper endoscopy (EGD)
- colonoscopy
- sigmoidoscopy

When you visit the doctor, bring any pictures taken during the procedure, as well as a copy of the *endoscopist's report*. If biopsies were taken during the endoscopy, bring a copy of the *biopsy report*. Most pediatric gastroenterologists will want to review the actual biopsy slides. The GI specialist who performed the endoscopy will not have the slides. You should request them from the pathology department at the center where the procedures were performed. That department may wish to mail the slides directly to the pediatric gastroenterologist or to the pa-

thology department in the hospital where the gastroenterologist works.

F. If your child has had any surgeries related to her digestive tract
problems, bring copies of the operative report and the pathology
report and slides (see discussion on procedures above).

G. Just prior to the visit, collect a stool sample from your child to
bring with you to the visit. One convenient way is to collect the
stool directly into a gallon-size food-storage bag and double-bag it.

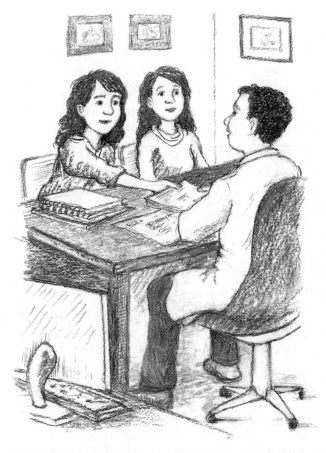

If your child has been evaluated at another hospital, it is helpful to give your
pediatric gastroenterologist copies of medical records, x-rays, endoscopy pictures, and pathology reports from the other facility.

Step 3. Write down a list of all the immediate concerns and any questions you and your child have.

- Bring this list with you to the first visit. If you don't bring a list, it's far too easy to forget your questions once the visit starts.

Preparing for Follow-Up Visits to the Gastroenterologist

Preparation always helps things go more smoothly and helps with treatment decisions. Be sure to prepare for subsequent visits to the doctor, too. Ask your child to keep a diary of her symptoms, starting one to two weeks before the next scheduled follow-up visit. This diary should include everything from Step 1 above. Ask your child to include the same level of detail about these symptoms as you did for the initial visit. Just in case it is needed, consider bringing a stool sample to this visit as well. (Your child's doctor may request it.)

Bring a list of all current medications, vitamins, and herbal supplements to the follow-up visit. Be prepared to discuss how and when your child is taking the medicines. If your child has any difficulties with taking any medicines, be honest with the doctor about this issue. Make notes beforehand of any side effects you or your child is noticing. For example, some medications can cause a rash, headaches, moodiness, or a puffy face.

Once again, write down all your questions and concerns before the visit. Bring the list with you.

Your gastroenterology health care team recognizes and appreciates the time and effort involved in thoroughly preparing for visits to their office. Your efforts will greatly enhance their ability to provide the best custom care for your child.

Helpful Dos and Don'ts for Any Visit

With the best of intentions, parents sometimes do things (or don't do things) that make the visit to the doctor more stressful for the child. Bear the following points in mind:

- Please do not promise your child that there will be no blood tests.
- Please do not look distressed when a rectal exam is done. A rectal exam involves looking at your child's bottom and sometimes probing inside with a gloved finger. This exam is often the best way to determine whether a child is in a flare. Although a rectal examination is not necessarily performed at every visit, it is sometimes needed for the doctor or nurse to provide the best care.
- Please do not look surprised when a doctor or nurse asks a child who is 13 or older to report the names and amounts of each medication he is taking. This is often the first step in helping him gain more independence and take charge of his inflammatory bowel disease.
- Unless otherwise instructed by the office of the pediatric gastroenterologist, please *do* let your child eat prior to the visit. Procedures are seldom performed on the day of the first visit or on a follow-up visit unless a plan that includes procedures is discussed beforehand with the parent.

❧ 6
Office Visits and Procedures for Children with IBD

Diagnosing IBD in a child, whether it is Crohn disease or ulcerative colitis, generally involves a series of steps. The diagnosis will proceed from the basic medical interview and physical examination to simple stool tests and blood tests and, when necessary, to x-rays and endoscopic tests (see chapter 9) requiring sedation or anesthesia. Only when the doctor strongly suspects that the child has IBD will she suggest invasive tests, such as a colonoscopy. Severely ill children may have to enter the hospital so that doctors can run tests more quickly and so that the children can be supported better during testing.

The Medical History Interview

The first step in making the diagnosis of IBD is the medical interview of the patient and family. The doctor asks whether the child has typical symptoms (diarrhea, rectal bleeding, and abdominal cramping). The doctor then tries to assess the severity of the symptoms, how long they have been present, and whether they are getting worse. To do this, the doctor obviously has to ask questions about body functions that are usually private. Although discussing bowel movements may be embarrassing for your child, these questions are extremely important.

The doctor will also ask questions to find out how the disease has affected your child's overall health. For example, has your child had fever, a low energy level, weight loss, or delays in growth or puberty?

Another critical part of the interview reviews other organs in the body, to assess whether *extraintestinal symptoms* (IBD symptoms that appear outside the digestive tract) are present.

The doctor's job is not only to assess whether your child's symptoms agree with the diagnosis of IBD, but also to reject the diagnoses of other disorders that can have similar symptoms (see chapters 3 and 4). The interview also includes a review of medical history such as previous surgeries or hospitalizations, family history (illness that may run in the family), and social history (where and with whom the child lives, school attendance). The medical history helps the doctor find out whether your child has other medical problems that might affect the diagnosis or treatment of colitis. Reviewing the family history is crucial, because as many as 30 percent of children with inflammatory bowel disease have close relatives with the disease. The social history is important to help the doctor understand how the disease is affecting school attendance and other activities.

The Physical Examination

The next step in the evaluation is a complete physical examination. This usually starts with measurement of height and weight so that the child's growth and nutritional status can be assessed. The doctor examines the child's skin, checking for paleness that might suggest anemia (low level of red blood cells). The doctor also checks the skin for the rashes that may accompany ulcerative colitis.

The oral examination is an important component of the physical exam. The doctor will look for mouth sores, which can be found in people with IBD, especially with Crohn disease. The heart and lungs are listened to. The abdomen is carefully examined for tenderness, swelling, enlargement of internal organs (such as the liver and spleen), and the presence of masses that might indicate areas of inflamed bowel.

The doctor will check the anal area for other causes of bleeding such as hemorrhoids or *fissures* (cracks in the skin), and for lesions typical of Crohn disease. A rectal examination (which requires the doctor to gently insert a gloved finger into the anus) may reveal a polyp or other abnormalities. During the rectal exam, a small stool sample may be obtained so that the laboratory can test for the presence of blood. The joints are examined for evidence of redness, pain, or swelling. Examination of the genitals to determine the stage of sexual maturity is important, since children with inflammatory bowel disease often enter puberty late.

Laboratory Tests

If the history and physical examination suggest that the child may have IBD, laboratory tests are done. (Laboratory tests are often called "studies.") Blood tests can help look for evidence of blood loss, inflammation, or nutritional deficiencies, and stool tests can identify infection. Additional blood tests can check how well other organs, such as the kidney and liver, are working. A urinalysis (urine test) is also helpful to check kidney function. These tests are described in more detail in chapter 7.

Imaging Studies

Radiographic studies can be important in the diagnosis of IBD. Plain x-rays of the abdomen can provide general information regarding the health of the intestine and can assess whether a complication, such as a blockage or perforation (hole), has occurred. X-ray studies that use contrast liquid (either swallowed or administered rectally) can give a "big picture" view of the anatomy of the intestines. These tests are described in more detail in chapter 8.

Endoscopic Evaluation

The most valuable studies to help make the diagnosis of IBD are endoscopic procedures that use long steerable tubes with a video chip on their end. The video component allows the doctor to examine the appearance of the internal lining of the upper and lower intestinal tracts. The doctors can also perform biopsies during these procedures. Biopsies involve taking small "pinch" samples of the lining of the intestine for later examination under a microscope. These tests are described in more detail in chapter 9.

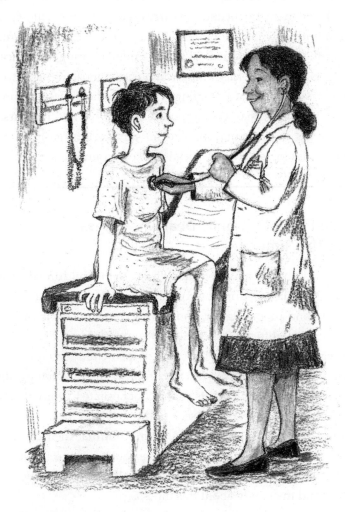

Physical examinations are part of the routine monitoring of children with Crohn disease or ulcerative colitis.

What Happens after My Child Has Been Diagnosed with IBD?

A diagnosis of IBD is difficult for both the child and the family. IBD is a chronic and unpredictable disease characterized by periods of disease remission interspersed with disease relapses. It is usually difficult to predict when a relapse might occur. Fortunately, most children respond well to treatment and can carry on with a normal lifestyle. All children with IBD need long-term follow-up by a gastroenterology team for the purpose of medical treatment, monitoring of medication side effects, treating disease complications, and most important, emotional support in the face of living with a chronic disease. In smaller practices, the team may be composed of a doctor and his nurse. In larger centers, the team may involve different doctors (gastroenterologist, endocrinologist), nurses, social workers, counselors, and a nutritionist.

How Do I Help My Family Deal with Stress during This Time?

The diagnosis of IBD may be difficult for both the child and the family. Having blood drawn, drinking contrast liquid (barium for an imaging studying), and preparing for, and having, an endoscopic procedure can certainly be difficult, especially for young children.

For parents, not knowing the cause of their child's symptoms, and experiencing the fear surrounding a chronic or life-threatening illness, may be overwhelming. Parents should not hesitate to voice their concerns to the medical team and seek additional help for themselves, if necessary. Although no one wants to find out that their child has a chronic disease, making the diagnosis has positive aspects. Diagnosis is the first step in starting treatment, and it allows for the education of the child and the family about this illness.

To help you and your family understand and accept the diagnosis of IBD, your child's doctor needs to be aware of how your family works. The doctor needs to know, for example, who the primary care-giver of the sick child will be (or whether there will be more than one primary caregiver). The primary caregiver will be the person who fills prescriptions, gives the child medications, and makes sure that the child gets to all of the follow-up appointments.

The sick child's siblings need to learn about IBD. It is an unfortu-nate fact that doctors, and even parents, often ignore siblings when bad things happen. Involving siblings when they are at an appropri-ate age has several good results. First, it ensures constant communica-tion between all family members, and thus the family works better as a unit. Second, it tends to make the child with IBD less different—the child is not singled out over his or her siblings. The third advantage is that including siblings avoids them feeling left out. Siblings of a child with IBD often feel isolated.

For most people and most ages, having information and knowing what to expect reduces anxiety, allows the child and family to feel more in control of the disease, and makes it possible for the family to work with the health care providers as a team.

When surveyed, teenagers with IBD say it is very important for the doctor to take time when giving them information about the diagnosis of IBD. These teenagers feel that the doctor should not appear rushed when giving them the information. They are also virtually unanimous in saying that they prefer having the doctor talk directly to them about IBD, rather than talking to them through their parents. In that direct communication process, they want the doctor to provide easy-to-understand information about the disease and what to expect.

Some parents prefer to hear the news of this diagnosis first so that they can help their children understand. The doctor will want to es-tablish a good relationship with every member of the family and dis-cuss the diagnosis and management of IBD in a way that works well for all of them.

Regardless of where you hear the diagnosis (in the doctor's office or in the recovery room, for example), take the time to let the informa-tion sink in, and be sure your doctor answers any questions you have.

The discussion should take place privately, not in a hallway outside the child's hospital room. You should also let your doctor know if you are too tired or stressed to receive the news. If you (or your child) do not feel you can handle any news at the moment, ask the doctor to talk to you a little later.

The doctor should discuss certain specific issues with you and your child when giving the diagnosis of IBD. She may not address all these concerns at the first visit, but she should cover them all within the first few visits after the diagnosis.

- The doctor should give the family information about important features of the disease, particularly definitions of IBD, Crohn disease, and ulcerative colitis.
- The doctor should tell the family who the members of the health care team are, what their roles are, and how to reach them.
- The doctor and the health care team should address the family's concerns and fears and answer their questions in a way that helps the parents and the child feel they have good control over the disease.

Most patients who are old enough and their families have several key concerns when they learn the diagnosis of IBD (see chapters 14–18). Usually these concerns involve the following:

- fear of hospitals, medications, and surgery
- the effect of IBD on school participation or participation in other activities
- fear of accidents at school or in other public places, and concern about inability to play with friends outside the home
- a child's feeling that the disease was his fault, and that he is a burden on others
- feeling isolated or "different"

If your child's doctor does not address these concerns, be sure to ask the doctor about them.

❧ 7
Laboratory Testing

Routine and specialized laboratory tests are regularly used to help make the diagnosis of and manage IBD. (These tests were mentioned in chapter 3 and will be discussed here in more detail.) Some tests are helpful in telling the difference between IBD and other conditions that have similar symptoms. Others can be used to tell the difference between Crohn disease and ulcerative colitis. Tests can also help doctors evaluate how active the disease is, or watch for disease-related complications or side effects of treatments. Test results are generally not used by themselves but are taken together with the overall condition and symptoms of the individual patient.

Laboratory Tests

IBD activity is usually monitored based on overall signs and symptoms such as whether the patient is having abdominal pain, diarrhea, blood in the stool, weight loss, or poor weight gain. The activity of the disease is also monitored by assessing the child's well-being in areas such as energy and activity levels, school attendance, and participation in sports and social functions.

Laboratory tests are helpful in disease management, too, because inflammation produces changes that can be measured in the blood and in the stool. Laboratory test results usually return to normal when the IBD is not active. Once disease-related blood and stool test results are known for a particular child (called baseline results), changes in those specific results can generally be used to monitor the activity of the child's IBD. Test results offer a way of assessing whether your child's IBD is active or inactive in addition to how she is acting and feeling.

Laboratory test results, which are not dependent on the child's understanding or opinion of the disease, can be particularly helpful in making treatment decisions about children and teenagers who are reluctant to discuss their symptoms. They are also helpful in children who feel well and have few, if any, symptoms but who still have considerable continuing intestinal inflammation.

Routine lab tests are usually ordered because they

- can help distinguish between IBD and noninflammatory conditions that have similar symptoms;
- provide a sense of how severe the inflammation is; and
- allow the doctor to identify which of the blood tests will be useful to follow, in order to monitor disease activity in this child.

Routine Blood Analysis

The results of routine blood tests generally show the following changes from the normal baseline when inflammation is active:

- white blood cell count (WBC) increases
- platelet count (Plt) increases
- erythrocyte sedimentation rate (ESR) increases
- C-reactive protein (CRP) increases
- red blood cell count (RBC) decreases (commonly referred to as anemia); the two most common measures of red blood cell numbers are the hemoglobin (Hgb) and hematocrit (Hct)
- albumin (one of the main blood proteins) decreases

Not all patients have all these abnormalities, and some patients may have normal or near-normal blood test values even though they still have very active IBD. It is also important to recognize that these blood tests are not specific for IBD. They may be abnormal in the face of *any* condition that causes inflammation, including infection.

Stool Studies

Stool culture, microscopic examination, and special testing of the stool all check for potential digestive tract infections. The presence of tiny amounts of blood in the stool is a nonspecific marker that may mean inflammation. Similarly, identification of elevated levels of the blood protein alpha-1-antitrypsin in the stool may be a sign of injury to the intestinal lining (this protein is resistant to the normal process of protein digestion in the gut). The presence of intact white blood cells in the stool also means inflammation, either from IBD or from infection in the gut. The presence of lactoferrin or calprotectin (types of proteins) in the stool is a marker of intestinal inflammation. Unfortunately, as with the routine blood tests, these stool tests are nonspecific and do not necessarily distinguish between intestinal inflammation caused by a bacterial infection and inflammation due to IBD.

Lab Tests to Monitor for Side Effects and Complications

Many of the blood tests used to track disease activity also provide information about potential medication-related side effects. These tests include blood counts and blood tests of how well the liver works (ALT, AST, GGT, bilirubin, alkaline phosphatase). Other important blood tests that check for treatment-related side effects are kidney function tests (BUN and creatinine) and tests of the pancreas (amylase and lipase). Nutritional deficiencies associated with IBD that can be detected through laboratory tests are vitamin levels, such as vitamin D or B_{12}, and levels of minerals such as zinc and iron.

The usefulness and potential harm of some IBD medications can be related to levels of the drug or to its breakdown products in the person's blood. Checking blood levels is important for the following medicines:

- cyclosporine
- tacrolimus

- 6-mercaptopurine (6-MP)
- azathioprine

Measuring drug levels or the levels of breakdown products can help doctors evaluate whether specific symptoms are due to side effects of the drug or to ongoing disease activity. Measuring drug levels can also help assess whether the child is taking the correct dose of the medication. It can identify whether a child may be having problems with drug absorption or with compliance (taking the medicine as directed). Constant disease activity despite the right drug levels in the blood may be a sign that the particular treatment is not effective for the child. The family and the doctor may want to explore different treatments rather than wait weeks or months to see what happens. It is possible to test a child ahead of time to find out whether he is able to break down 6-MP and azathioprine; if he is not, then different medications will be more effective for that child.

IBD-Specific Laboratory Tests

Antibodies are proteins that the immune system produces to fight infections and unfamiliar material that enters the body. When antibodies fight infections, they cause inflammation. The search for the trigger of the typical abnormal inflammation in IBD has led to the discovery of several specific antibodies. These antibodies are present in the blood of many people with Crohn disease or ulcerative colitis but are usually not present in children without IBD. The most commonly identified markers are pANCA and ASCA. Newer antibody tests have also been developed: anti-outer membrane protein C (OmpC) and anti-CBir1.

As we have discussed and as you may know first hand, diagnosing pediatric IBD is challenging. This is why the search for accurate, noninvasive markers of IBD has been stepped up. These antibody markers, when they are found in diagnostic test results, may help doctors recognize IBD more quickly. They may also indicate whether a child has Crohn disease, ulcerative colitis, or some other condition. However, these laboratory tests are *not* specific for IBD. At times, the detected levels may be falsely elevated in normal people (false positive). Other times, the results may be negative when a child actually has IBD. Therefore, these blood tests are *not* a substitute for x-rays and colonoscopy.

The IBD marker tests involve only blood tests, and they do not require putting a scope or other instrument inside the body. Talk with your child's doctor about whether antibody tests can be helpful in your child's particular case. Future research will focus on identifying more of these antibodies to improve our ability to diagnose IBD with confidence.

8 Imaging Studies

This chapter describes some of the imaging studies used most often to diagnose IBD and to monitor its potential complications. Imaging studies use x-rays, sound waves, or other methods to take pictures of the inside of the body.

Abdominal Plain Film

The abdominal plain film is a simple x-ray picture of the abdomen (belly area), taken when your child is either lying flat on the x-ray table or standing up. This picture can show how much air and stool is in the intestine. The pattern of air and stool can be helpful in showing whether your child is constipated. The doctor can also learn from this x-ray whether there might be a blockage or a hole in the intestine.

This type of x-ray is sometimes called the KUB, which stands for kidney-ureter-bladder. The x-ray is supposed to include the kidneys, ureters (the tubes that go from the kidneys to the bladder), and the bladder, but in reality these three organs usually do not show well on the abdominal plain film.

Upper Gastrointestinal (GI) and Small Bowel Series

The upper GI and small bowel series are x-ray pictures of the abdomen performed after the patient drinks liquid barium. *Barium* is a type of chemical that tastes a little like chalk, but sometimes the taste can be improved by adding chocolate or strawberry flavoring to the liquid. Still, many children find drinking the barium difficult, and they often require some coaxing. On x-ray, the barium shows up white, while the rest of the body is mostly gray or black.

The contrast of white as it goes through the digestive tract gives a picture of the size, shape, and location of

- the esophagus (the tube leading from the throat to the stomach),
- the stomach, and
- the small intestine.

This test shows pictures of what the inside of the digestive tract looks like, but it does not show the actual lining and muscles of the tract. The test is generally normal in ulcerative colitis, but it can show changes in the small intestine that would suggest Crohn disease. The test is useful in detecting a shaggy lining or separation of parts of the intestine. Shaggy linings and separations can indicate swelling and irritation.

The upper gastrointestinal and small bowel series can also show other problems:

- ulceration
- narrowing (stricture) in the small intestine
- an enlarged intestinal segment that could mean there is a blockage
- a fistula (an abnormal connection between loops of the intestine)

This study typically requires fasting (nothing by mouth) for about four hours before the test. Since the goal of the test is to examine the entire small intestine, the procedure may take three hours or longer (with periods of x-raying alternating with periods of waiting). At some point, the radiologist may push on the child's abdomen to help separate the loops of intestine to achieve better x-ray pictures.

Barium Enema

The barium enema is an x-ray of the colon (the large intestine). The barium is squirted up into the rectum (which connects the colon to the anus) through a tube inserted into the anal opening. Under pressure, the barium goes through the entire colon, all the way to its beginning (called the cecum). The white barium gives a picture of the size, shape, and appearance of the colon. It outlines what the inside of the colon looks like but does not make a picture of the actual lining and muscles of the colon. This test is useful in detecting a shaggy lining (which would indicate swelling and irritation).

The barium enema can also show other problems:

- ulceration
- narrowing (stricture) in the small intestine
- an enlarged intestinal segment that could mean there is a blockage
- a fistula (an abnormal connection between loops of the intestine)

Sometimes the barium goes into the terminal ileum, the part of the small intestine that connects to the colon. When this happens, the doctors can see that area as well. Although the barium enema used to be a common test in patients with suspected IBD, it is rarely needed now that colonoscopies (see chapter 9) are widely performed in children.

Computed Tomography

Computed tomography, or CT scan—sometimes referred to as a CAT scan—is a special kind of x-ray that converts computer images of the body into pictures. In this test, the patient drinks a large amount of a special liquid dye (called an *oral contrast*) that helps show the size, shape, and location of the GI tract. Usually, the radiologist also injects a different contrast material into the veins (*IV contrast*). IV contrast shows more clearly the features of the solid organs (like the liver and kidneys). The patient lies inside a short cylinder that houses a camera, which takes pictures from different angles. The camera usually makes noise as it moves inside the cylinder.

A CT scan of the abdomen and pelvis, with oral and IV contrast dyes, can provide a great deal of information about the GI tract, including

- the presence of an abscess (a pocket of infection)
- the possibility of appendicitis
- whether the bowel wall is too thick (indicating the presence of swelling and irritation of the intestine)
- a narrow or enlarged segment of bowel
- a fistula (an abnormal connection between loops of the intestine)

The CT scan shows pictures of the lining and muscles of the GI tract as well as some pictures of the inside of the tract. Other solid organs, including the liver, spleen, gallbladder, pancreas, and kidneys, are also visible on the CT scan. The test further shows normal and abnormal lymph nodes, and tumors in the abdomen.

Ultrasound

The ultrasound uses sound waves to make images, much like a submarine uses sonar to make a picture of the bottom of the ocean. The sound waves are aimed at, and bounce off, the intestines and other organs in the abdomen. These organs include the gallbladder, pancreas, kidneys, and appendix. The patient does not have to drink any contrast dye or have anything put in the rectum. No intravenous (IV) liquids are necessary. A technician will spread a gel over the abdomen, and the ultrasound device painlessly touches the skin, sliding over the gel.

The ultrasound shows the appearance of the muscles of the digestive tract but not the inside of the tract. This test is useful in detecting gallstones, pancreatitis, kidney stones, or kidney blockage. The test can also point to the possibility of appendicitis, and show whether the bowel wall is thick and swollen, possibly as a result of inflammation.

Magnetic Resonance Imaging

A magnetic resonance imaging (MRI) test uses magnets to excite molecules (tiny particles) in the cells of the body. In people with digestive system problems (such as IBD), the MRI is used to evaluate the liver

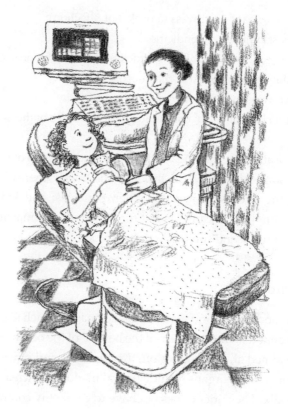

Diagnostic imaging of children with IBD sometimes involves doing an ultrasound of the abdomen.

and the pancreas, but it is not very good at showing the intestines. MRI does not expose the patient to any harmful radiation. During the test, the patient lies inside a long tube with magnets moving noisily around the body. Sometimes contrast material is injected into the veins to produce better pictures.

Some patients feel uncomfortable while inside the tube, because they do not like being enclosed in a tight space. Many young children receive sedation (medicine to make them sleepy) before an MRI test. Sedation makes children feel more comfortable, and allows them to hold still for the test.

Bone Age X-Ray

The bone age x-ray evaluates how mature the child's bones are and how much more growing they are able to do. The bones of the hands and wrists in children have growth centers that develop and then disappear into the bones. Bones look different as the child ages and then when the bones are fully grown. The bone age x-ray compares the age of the bones with the age of your child. When the bone age is less than your child's age, there is more time for the bones to keep growing. A short child who has a bone age less than the child's age is likely to keep growing and has the potential to catch up and grow to the height that she was meant to be based on her genes.

Bone Density Scan

A bone density scan, also called dual-energy x-ray absorptiometry (DEXA), is a special form of x-ray technology that measures bone mineral density and that is used to diagnose low bone density (osteopenia or osteoporosis). Decreased bone density is common in adults with IBD and can be seen in children and adolescents with IBD as well. Considerably decreased bone density can increase the risk of broken bones (fractures).

Poor nutrition, low vitamin and mineral levels, little exercise or weightbearing activities, or use of corticosteroids (such as prednisone) can increase the risk of low bone density. The bone density scan uses a very small dose of radiation and is most often performed on the lower spine and hips. The patient lies on a table that has an "arm" suspended overhead. The test is painless and takes 10 or 15 minutes.

Tests for Special Purposes

Newly developed imaging tests can help in the diagnosis of inflammatory bowel disease and its related complications. This section will highlight three such techniques. These techniques now make it possible to see areas that were previously only reachable through invasive endoscopic procedures (see chapter 9), or through surgical exploration. These special imaging procedures are becoming more common as doctors seek noninvasive ways of evaluating patients. None of these methods, however, gives doctors the opportunity to take biopsies (tissue samples for examination) or to treat strictures (narrowed areas in the intestines).

Capsule Endoscopy

Beyond the first part of the small intestine (the duodenum), and near the last part (the terminal ileum), the rest of the small intestine (8 to 16 feet) is usually impossible to reach with a standard endoscope. Wireless capsule endoscopy is a technique of viewing the entire small intestine with a video camera housed in a small pill (a pill camera) that is about one inch long and half an inch wide. The patient can swallow the capsule, or the doctor can place it in the small intestine using an endoscope. The video capsule is equipped with a camera and an eight-hour battery.

The capsule is able to transmit continuous video images as it travels through the small intestine. A receiver captures and stores these images. The information is then downloaded into a computer equipped with specialized software, which allows the doctor to see the lining of the entire small intestine. Inflamed areas, ulcers, bleeding lesions, pseudopolyps (inflamed tissue that looks like polyps), or even narrowed areas can be identified. Because the patient is wearing multiple circular patches (receivers) over the entire abdomen, the position of these abnormal areas can be pinpointed, and pictures or even video clips can be stored for later examination. The capsule is expelled in a bowel movement and flushed down the toilet.

Magnetic Resonance Cholangiopancreatography

Some patients with IBD develop inflammation and strictures in their bile ducts, inside and outside the liver. This condition is called *primary sclerosing cholangitis* (PSC). PSC normally occurs after the diagnosis of IBD is made, though it sometimes exists before it is known that the child has IBD. Up until a decade ago, the only way to diagnose PSC was through an endoscopy in which a catheter was inserted into the bile ducts. This invasive procedure is called *endoscopic retrograde cholangiopancreatography* (ERCP).

Over the last ten years, examination of the bile ducts inside and outside the liver has been perfected using a special noninvasive imaging technique called magnetic resonance cholangiopancreatography (MRCP). MRCP takes advantage of the fact that structures filled with nonmoving or slow-moving fluids, such as bile ducts, appear bright white against a black background in an MRI. This circumstance often makes it unnecessary to perform the more invasive ERCP study. As with regular MRI tests, some children will need sedation for the MRCP.

Virtual Colonoscopy

Improvements in CT techniques, and the use of computer modeling, have allowed radiologists to reconstruct a 3-D model of the colon, called a *CT colonography* (or, more popularly, virtual colonoscopy). In adults, the procedure takes about 10 minutes and requires no sedation. Patients lie on their backs while a continuously rotating x-ray beam provides images of the entire colon. The procedure is repeated with the patient on his stomach. A computer program puts these images together in a movielike series of 3-D pictures.

This technique is most useful in detecting colon polyps and screening for colon cancer. At this point, not many studies apply CT colonography to the diagnosis of inflammatory bowel disease. Strictures and wall thickening indicating diffuse inflammation may be detected using this technique, but flat lesions and the shallow ulcerations that characterize IBD may not be detected by this method. With continued improvements in resolution and speed, both CT-based and MRI-based computer modeling will likely find greater uses in diagnosing and monitoring children with inflammatory bowel disease.

✥ 9

Endoscopic Exams

Endoscopy of the digestive tract is a tool that most people with IBD are or will become familiar with. It is one of the most commonly used tools to diagnose IBD. Endoscopy involves the use of a specially designed camera called an endoscope to look inside the intestines. Doctors use endoscopy to diagnose IBD and to help them determine and monitor the treatment of the disease. The special camera allows doctors to see areas of the digestive tract that may be inflamed in patients with IBD or similar conditions. It also allows doctors to detect other types of inflammation, such as those caused by excessive stomach acid (reflux), bacterial or viral infections, or medications. This chapter describes the procedures, including how to prepare for them and what's involved in the recovery period.

Types of Endoscopic Procedures

Four main types of endoscopy are performed in pediatric patients with IBD (figure 9.1).

1. Upper endoscopy, or EGD (esophagogastroduodenoscopy), examines the esophagus, stomach, and upper portions of the small intestine.
2. Colonoscopy looks at the entire colon (large intestine) and often the last part of the small intestine (terminal ileum).
3. Sigmoidoscopy is a special, limited form of colonoscopy. It examines only the last two parts of the colon: the rectum (the very end of the colon) and the sigmoid colon (the portion of the colon

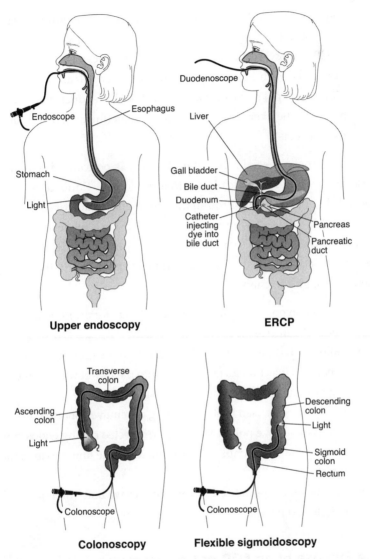

Figure 9.1. Endoscopic procedures in inflammatory bowel disease. In upper endoscopy, a long flexible tube is passed into the mouth and is used to examine the esophagus, stomach, and upper small intestine (*top left*). A modified version of this procedure, called endoscopic retrograde cholangiopancreatography (ERCP), can be used to evaluate the bile ducts and pancreas (*top right*). Lower GI endoscopy is done by inserting a tube through the anus and examining the entire colon (colonoscopy, *bottom left*) or a portion of the colon (sigmoidoscopy, *bottom right*).

just above the rectum). Sigmoidoscopy typically requires less sedation and less preparation than a full colonoscopy.

4. ERCP (endoscopic retrograde cholangiopancreatography) is
   performed with a specially designed endoscope (called a side-
   viewing scope) that can evaluate the bile ducts (ducts that drain
   bile from the liver) and the pancreatic duct (the duct that drains
   the pancreas).

Each of these special types of endoscopy is performed with an endoscope designed specifically for that procedure. Endoscopes have a
special channel running through them that allows doctors to wash the
bowel or blow in air to improve their view during the test. This channel also allows doctors to pass instruments in and out during the procedure. A pediatric gastroenterologist might pass any of these instruments through the channel:

- biopsy forceps, to obtain a sample of tissue for examination
  under the microscope
- balloons that can dilate (widen) narrowed areas of the bowel
- needles to inject medicine directly into the bowel wall, including medicine to help control bleeding
- various probes used to stop bleeding or remove abnormal tissue
- snares to remove polyps that may be detected during endoscopy
- brushes that can sample fluid or mucus on the lining to look for
  infections
- various other specialized forceps, to retrieve both foreign
  objects and polyps

The Purpose of an EGD or Colonoscopy

Children and adolescents with IBD usually need an endoscopy for
one or more of these six reasons:

1. to confirm a diagnosis of IBD
2. to evaluate (or reevaluate) how much of the bowel is sick, and
   how severely it is affected

3. to help the physician determine whether a change in treatment is needed
4. to treat symptoms or complications of IBD, such as bleeding
5. to treat a specific problem—for example, to widen a stricture (narrow area)
6. to look for precancerous changes

Biopsies are taken from all segments of the colon and are very important in deciding whether the condition is ulcerative colitis, Crohn disease, or colitis due to infection. Biopsies are also important in assessing the severity of the inflammation. In long-standing disease (ten years' duration or more), biopsies done during a colonoscopy can detect the early changes of colon cancer.

Having a colonoscopy may be uncomfortable, even painful, because the colonoscope is pushed around the turns in the large intestine. The bloating that results from filling the colon with air (so the doctor can see the lining) adds to the discomfort. Children who know they will be having the procedure are often anxious and frightened, and therefore colonoscopy is usually performed under heavy sedation given through an IV, or under general anesthesia.

Doctors and parents understand how important it is to make this procedure as pain-free as possible for children with ulcerative colitis, because they will certainly need another colonoscopy as the years go by. Younger children as well as anxious teenagers and young adults are given general anesthesia by an anesthesiologist. For older, cooperative, and less anxious children, a technique called conscious sedation is used. In conscious sedation, the child is given medication to make him sleepy and comfortable during the procedure, but an anesthesiologist is not present. The medication for conscious sedation is usually administered by the gastroenterologist and nurses performing the procedure.

Most people who have had a colonoscopy agree that the most difficult part of the process is preparing the colon before the procedure. The purpose of the colon preparation is to remove fecal material (stool) from the colon so that the lining of the large intestine can be examined effectively. Preparation can be done in different ways (see below), but there is no easy way to clean out the colon. When cleaning cannot be done successfully at home, it may have to be done in the hospital. Procedures may be canceled and rescheduled if the clean-out is not adequate.

Parents need to understand the options for preparing the bowel and sedating their child. Discussing these options with the doctor will minimize stress and ensure that the special needs of the child are met.

Although colonoscopy is generally a very safe procedure, there are known risks, including inadvertently putting a hole in the colon (perforation), or causing additional bleeding or an infection. In addition, the sedation or anesthesia itself carries a small risk of side effects. It is the responsibility of the colonoscopist to explain these risks to the family, and to obtain their written consent for the procedure. The consent form indicates that the risks of the procedure have been discussed with the parent.

How Is Endoscopy Done in Children and Adolescents with IBD?

Doctors with special training in pediatric gastroenterology, including pediatric endoscopy, perform the procedure. As noted above, to minimize discomfort, patients are usually under some form of sedation or anesthesia (deeply relaxed or sleeping).

In EGD and ERCP, the endoscope passes through the mouth into the esophagus (the pipe that takes food from the throat into the stomach), and from the esophagus into the stomach and the small intestine. Standard upper endoscopes can pass only into the first portion of the small intestine, known as the duodenum. An additional 19 to 26 feet (6 to 8 meters) of small intestine are not reachable by standard upper endoscopy. The doctor may use a longer endoscope, an enteroscope, to examine the second part of the small intestine, known as the jejunum, especially for patients who are thought to have small bowel disease farther down in the intestine. In ERCP, which usually involves injecting a special dye into the bile or pancreatic ducts, the endoscope passes into the second portion of the duodenum, where the bile and pancreatic ducts drain into the bowel.

In colonoscopy and sigmoidoscopy, the endoscope enters through the anus into the rectum and from there passes throughout the remainder of the colon. The colon is a long and winding organ shaped something like a question mark, measuring 3 to 6 feet (1 to 2 meters) in an adult. Colonoscopy is more difficult to perform than an EGD and often takes somewhat longer.

During a colonoscopy in patients with known or suspected IBD, most pediatric gastroenterologists attempt to enter the very end of the small intestine, known as the terminal ileum. Because the terminal ileum is the portion of the bowel that is commonly involved with Crohn disease, examining this area is important when trying to distinguish between ulcerative colitis and Crohn disease.

Preparation and Procedure

Most endoscopic examinations are elective rather than emergency procedures, which means that the doctor, patient, and family are able to schedule the procedure. If elective, the procedure is performed when the patient is considered healthy. Patients (or their parents) should tell their doctors if illness symptoms develop before the procedure, such as a cough, runny nose, fever, or other problems. The doctor may want to reschedule the procedure for another day, to reduce the risk of complications, such as infection.

In some patients who are ill (either in the hospital or at home), the procedure may need to be performed despite the illness symptoms. For example, these exams may be needed to diagnose IBD, or to assist in the treatment of a patient who is becoming increasingly ill due to her IBD. The procedures may be necessary for the treatment of children with complications of IBD. Patients and their families should understand the possible increased risk connected with having these procedures done while the patient is ill. Discuss with the doctor any concerns you have.

EGD, ERCP, and Capsule Endoscopy

For most patients with IBD, the only required preparation for EGD, ERCP, and capsule endoscopy is fasting. The length of fasting is determined by the patient's age. You should check with your child's doctor for the appropriate fasting time for your child. If your child takes daily medications such as medicines for diabetes, seizures, or other chronic conditions, you should check with his doctor for specific instructions. Some medications should not be taken on the day of the procedure, and the dosage of some medicines may need to change on the day of the test. If your child has a heart condition or a prosthetic device, check with his doctor for specific instructions regarding preventive antibiotics before or after the procedure. Some patients who are having an ERCP will receive antibiotics before the procedure because they are at an increased risk of infection due to their underlying condition. Blood tests or x-rays may also be required before the procedure, if the doctor thinks they would be helpful.

Colonoscopy and Sigmoidoscopy

A colonoscopy requires fasting before the procedure as well as bowel clean-out before the procedure. The bowel is cleaned out for three reasons.

1. Bowel cleaning in advance allows the doctor to effectively examine the lining of the large intestine for abnormalities.
2. A clean bowel makes the procedure easier to perform.
3. A clean bowel reduces the risk of complications for the patient.

Doctors may choose to cancel the colonoscopy in a patient who has not had a good bowel cleaning. Although doctors have some ability to wash the bowel during the colonoscopy, this washing does not make up for an unprepared bowel.

Bowel-cleaning routines differ among medical centers and even among doctors at the same center. There are different routines because there is no one "best" method that works in all patients, that is easy to take, and that is completely effective. Bowel preparation usually includes taking in only clear liquids (water, clear broth, etc.) for one to two days before the procedure, and adding a laxative. A laxative is a medicine (prescription or over the counter) that encourages bowel movements. This medicine is given on the day of the procedure or two days prior to the procedure. Common medicines used for this purpose include polyethylene glycol, sodium phosphate-containing medicines, and magnesium-containing medications, such as magnesium citrate. Medicines are usually in liquid form, although some are available as pills. In addition, some doctors tell their patients to have enemas, either on the evening before or on the morning of the procedure. The specific bowel-cleaning procedure fits the patient's age and weight. A different procedure can be used if the first one does not work as expected. Even in patients who have diarrhea, a specific bowel-cleaning procedure is usually required.

Flexible sigmoidoscopy generally requires a modification of the colonoscopy routine outlined above. In some patients who are having significant diarrhea, additional bowel-cleansing medications are not required for a flexible sigmoidoscopy. If patients will be sedated for the procedure, fasting beforehand is necessary.

Sedation and Anesthesia

There are many types of sedation that a child can receive for the endoscopic procedure. Medicines for sedation reduce discomfort during the exam and make the child forget the experience when it is over. Doctors generally group the level of sedation a patient will get into one of three categories: conscious sedation, deep sedation, or general anesthesia.

Patients receiving conscious sedation are able to respond to commands during the procedure but generally do not remember the procedure or experience pain during it. Patients who are under deep sedation or general anesthesia cannot respond to commands, do not remember the procedure, and do not experience pain during it. Depending on the medicine used, however, patients under deep sedation or general an-

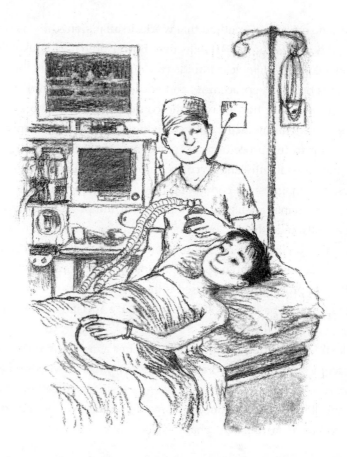

Patients undergoing upper endoscopy or colonoscopy are given sedation or anesthesia to keep them comfortable.

esthesia may take longer to wake up from the procedure than patients under conscious sedation. Patients who are under deep sedation or general anesthesia usually have an anesthesiologist involved in their procedure, which may increase the cost and time it takes.

What to Expect during the Procedure

Depending on the procedure, patients may lie on their back, on their left side, or, for ERCP, on their stomach. Patients undergoing an EGD under conscious sedation may experience some very brief gagging during the procedure. Most patients do not remember this. Those undergoing colonoscopy may experience abdominal cramping or distension (feeling full) during the procedure. This discomfort is due to the air the doctor blows into the bowel to help the scope pass and to help the doctor see the lining of the bowel. The doctor is able to remove some of the air when removing the scope at the conclusion of the colonoscopy, but the patient frequently needs to pass the air (pass gas) after the procedure is done. This will relieve the feeling of fullness or bloating.

Cramping can also occur during these procedures because the endoscope forms loops. Pediatric gastroenterologists are particularly aware of the discomfort associated with loop formation, and they try to minimize it if possible, but some looping can still occur. Patients may be turned to one side or the other during the procedure to help reduce looping. The cramping due to looping is usually short lived.

Biopsies are not painful. In fact, if a conscious patient were not told that a biopsy was being performed, she would probably not be able to tell when the biopsy was happening. Pain in the bowel is caused by distension, not from the small pinching that occurs during biopsies. Although patients and families are often most concerned about what biopsies will feel like, this part of the endoscopic procedure is usually the least uncomfortable.

The feeling of gagging (with upper endoscopy) or cramping (with lower endoscopy) usually improves when the scope is withdrawn in the second half of the endoscopic procedure. This is when treatment procedures such as biopsies or polyp removal are typically done.

What to Expect after the Procedure

EGD

Patients may be nauseated after an upper endoscopy and may have a sore throat. A few patients may need to be given intravenous (IV) fluids or an antinausea medication after the procedure. Generally, though, these problems go away with little treatment. Severe chest pain can develop after an upper endoscopy, and patients or family members should notify their doctor immediately if the patient develops significant chest pain after endoscopy, or if he has other symptoms as described below (under ERCP).

ERCP

Patients who have had an ERCP are at risk for complications after the procedure, including pancreatitis, infection with or without fever, and gastrointestinal bleeding if a treatment was performed during the procedure. Pancreatitis is usually associated with severe abdominal pain. Seek immediate medical attention if your child develops

- pain
- fever
- vomiting of blood
- blood in the stool or black stools
- dizziness or lightheadedness

Colonoscopy and Flexible Sigmoidoscopy

After the procedure, many patients experience some degree of nausea, fullness, or bloating. A few patients may need to be given IV fluids or an antinausea medication after the procedure. Generally, though, these problems disappear with little treatment. Patients who develop significant abdominal pain, increased blood in their bowel movements, or fever should seek immediate medical attention.

Procedures Performed under Sedation or General Anesthesia

In addition to infection, bleeding, and pain from the procedure, patients experience side effects from the anesthesia or sedation, or from the way it was given. (A side effect does not necessarily indicate a problem with the procedure or with the anesthesia, however.) Common side effects include sleepiness, nausea, and vomiting. If a patient had a breathing tube in her throat during the procedure, she may experience a sore throat for a few days. The patient is generally advised not to return to work or school on the day of an endoscopic procedure with sedation. Patients who are old enough to drive should not do so until the day after the procedure. Patients should not engage in activities that require a high degree of coordination until the next day, when the effects of anesthesia and sedation will have worn off.

Patients or their families should contact their doctors immediately after a procedure if any of the following symptoms develop:

- breathing difficulties
- chest or abdominal pain
- fever
- prolonged vomiting
- increased blood in the stool
- vomiting blood
- any other concerns

The above listing is not all inclusive. Ask the doctor for instructions regarding procedures before *and after* any endoscopy. If you are unable to contact the doctor and are concerned about symptoms that occur after the procedure, take your child to the emergency room for evaluation.

Risks and Complications of Endoscopy

As with any procedure, there are risks associated with endoscopy. If your child receives medications to sedate him on any level, there are also risks associated with these medications and the way they are given. We suggest that you and your family discuss the potential risks and complications with the doctors who will be performing the procedure and with the anesthesiologist, if an anesthesiologist will be part of the endoscopy.

The risks and potential complications of endoscopy include

- a hole in the intestinal tract (perforation)
- increased or new bleeding
- infection

- breathing problems
- a bad reaction to medication

The degree of risk varies depending on several factors, including

- the child's symptom
- how much of the bowel is affected by the disease
- the child's general health
- the type of procedure the child is having
- how well the bowel is cleaned out (for colonoscopy and flexible sigmoidoscopy)
- whether a more difficult procedure is being performed during the endoscopy (for example, dilating or stretching a portion of the bowel that is narrowed)

In general, the risk of a healthy and well-prepared patient experiencing some type of complication in a normal upper endoscopy or colonoscopy is between 1 in 1,000 cases to 1 in 10,000 cases. Endoscopic risk also depends on the experience of the doctor performing the test. Patients and their families should ask their doctor about her experience with pediatric endoscopy. Ideally the doctor has a great deal of experience and a very low complication rate.

Patients and families can help decrease the risk of complications by telling their doctors about any other medical problems the child has. Your child's doctor also needs to know about any prior problems your child has had with procedures or sedation as well as any related family medical history. Patients or caregivers should also alert the doctor if the patient develops illness symptoms such as cough, fever, and congestion prior to his scheduled procedure.

Patients must strictly follow the doctor's orders for preparations before the procedure, such as having nothing by mouth prior to the endoscopy. Patients who eat prior to an endoscopic procedure but are supposed to be fasting place themselves at risk for vomiting during the procedure. The vomitus may enter the airway and cause severe pneumonia. Maintaining strict preprocedure fasting is especially important in young children who, not understanding the potentially severe consequences, may try to sneak food. Similarly, failure to take the fully prescribed bowel preparation increases the difficulty of the procedure, makes it more likely that an important finding may be missed, prolongs the procedure, and increases the risk of complications, such as a perforation.

Pediatric gastrointestinal endoscopy is a developing field in which there have been significant advances in the last thirty years. There will be continued advances in this field in the years to come. Endoscopy and endoscopic biopsy are the standard tools for making the diagnosis of Crohn disease or ulcerative colitis at this time.

Patients with IBD will likely need more than one endoscopic procedure in their lifetime. Doctors and nurses are working with patients and their families to make these important procedures as safe and easy to tolerate as possible, while still keeping them useful. Endoscopic treatment procedures are also performed on children with IBD. In many cases, the availability of pediatric therapeutic endoscopy (treatments through endoscopy) has reduced the need for surgery in children with ulcerative colitis or Crohn disease.

Part III
Treating IBD

❦ 10
Medications

Although no current medications cure ulcerative colitis or Crohn disease, medications can provide a feeling of well-being that helps children lead normal daily lives. The goals of treatment are to bring the disease under control (induce remission) and keep it controlled (maintain remission). A trusting relationship between the child, the family, and the health care team is extremely important for achieving the goals of treatment.

Inducing and Maintaining Remission

Periods of increased disease activity (flares) are characteristic of IBD. A key goal in the treatment of IBD is finding effective *induction* treatment. Induction puts the disease into *remission*. When disease is in remission, the symptoms of the disease, such as diarrhea, pain, bleeding, poor appetite and tiredness, disappear. Nutritional status also improves, allowing for normal growth and the eventual attainment of normal pubertal development. The health care team can check whether the disease is active or in remission through physical exams, which include tracking growth and development, and by using laboratory testing when needed. In truth, you and your child will often know better than anyone else if the disease is active or not.

The first goal of treatment is to reach a point where the disease is not interfering with the child's daily activities or overall well-being. This is a very important concept. Too many children and their families accept the child feeling "okay, I guess." Feeling "okay, I guess" is not true remission!

After inducing remission, the next goal of treatment is to form a plan that will keep the disease in remission. This is the *maintenance* treatment. The ideal maintenance medication will ward off flares of disease with minimal side effects.

Medications Used for Treating IBD

Most of the medications prescribed for IBD may be used both for induction therapy and for maintenance therapy (table 10.1). Your physician will decide which of the medications to prescribe initially for your child depending on the severity of your child's symptoms. Medications can be administered orally (by mouth), intravenously (through a needle in the vein), by injection intramuscularly (a shot in the muscle) or injection subcutaneously (a shot under the skin), or rectally (by enema or suppository).

- Oral medications can exert their effects systemically if they are absorbed through the lining of the intestines into the bloodstream.
- Intravenous medications are injected into the bloodstream. They travel throughout the entire body to the inflamed bowel through the blood vessels serving the intestines.
- Other routes of injection, including shots into the muscles or under the skin, also deliver medications that work throughout the body (systemic).
- Since the lining of the gut is the site of the body affected in IBD, medications have also been designed that are active only when they are in contact with the inflamed lining of the gut. These targeted medications stay largely within the bowel and are poorly absorbed because of their chemical structures or coatings. Their special features allow them to target their effects to specific regions of the intestinal tract.

In this chapter, we describe IBD medications and treatments in the order in which they appear in table 10.1.

Table 10.1. Treatments for inducing and maintaining remission

	Induction	Maintenance
5-Aminosalicylates (5-ASA)	+	+
Corticosteroids	+	–
Immunomodulators	–	+
Biologics	+	+
Antibiotics	+	+
Nutrition	+	+

5-Aminosalicylates

The 5-aminosalicylate (5-ASA) drugs include some of the oldest medications used for inflammatory bowel disease. The generic names for these drugs are sulfasalazine, mesalamine, olsalazine, balsalazide. The brand names are Apriso, Azulfidine, Colazal, Dipentum, Asacol, Pentasa, Lialda, Salofalk, Rowasa, Canasa. These medications are anti-inflammatory medications that are chemically related to aspirin. Their anti-inflammatory effects are concentrated mostly in the bowel. There are rectal as well as oral formulations of salicylates. In addition, some preparations release the active drug at different levels of the small and large intestine. These options make it possible for your child's doctor to select the best preparation depending on which area of the bowel the disease is affecting. Studies, as well as clinical experience, show that these medications can be used for induction in patients who have mild disease. In addition, salicylates are safe and effective maintenance medications in ulcerative colitis, as well as in some patients with Crohn disease.

The 5-aminosalicylates are the mainstay of maintenance treatment in mild to moderate ulcerative colitis. When given by mouth, they can provide long-term remission. Suppositories deliver medication to the rectum, and enemas deliver the medicine to the lower part of the large intestine (left colon). These forms can be used long term or periodically for breakthrough symptoms.

5-ASA can also be used at times for long-term maintenance in mild to moderate Crohn disease. Oral preparations deliver the active medication to the small and large bowel. Therefore, these medications can

Table 10.2. Pill and rectal forms of the 5-Aminosalicylates

Most aminosalicylate medications are taken by mouth, and some of them are also available in enema or suppository form. This table lists the different forms of these medications.

Pill (oral tablet coatings)

Sustained release: Pentasa, Lialda
pH (acid) sensitive release: Salofalk, Asacol

Pill (bacterial enzyme [azoreductase] release)

Sulfasalazine: mesalamine linked to a weak sulfa antibiotic (sulfapyridine)
Balsalazide (Colazal): mesalamine linked to an inactive carrier molecule
Olsalazine (Dipentum): two mesalamine molecules linked together

Rectal

Rowasa
Pentasa rectal suspension or suppositories
Salofalk rectal suspension or suppositories
Canasa suppositories

be used for different disease locations. The different applications of various 5-ASA drugs are summarized in table 10.2 and described below.

5-Aminosalicylic Acid Formulations

Sulfasalazine (Azulfidine) was the first 5-ASA compound used successfully to treat ulcerative colitis and Crohn colitis. It is taken by mouth and is available in both coated and uncoated tablet forms. It can be made by the pharmacist into a liquid preparation for children who are unable to swallow tablets. About 25 percent of the drug is absorbed from the small intestine into the bloodstream. The remainder passes into the colon, where normal bacteria break down this medication into its two components, 5-ASA and sulfapyridine.

The sulfapyridine molecule acts only as a carrier to deliver the active portion, 5-ASA, to the colon. The sulfapyridine, which contains sulfa in its chemical structure, is responsible for most of the side effects caused by sulfasalazine (see below). Most of the medicine remains in contact with the inflamed lining of the colon. Eventually, the 5-ASA passes from the body in the stool.

Sulfasalazine in Ulcerative Colitis and Crohn Colitis/Ileocolitis

Virtually all data regarding the treatment of IBD with different types of 5-ASA are derived from adult experience. Sulfasalazine is often effective in mild-to-moderate active ulcerative colitis and Crohn colitis / ileocolitis. Symptoms of mild inflammation should disappear in 60 to 70 percent of patients within three to four weeks of starting treatment. Success rates with sulfasalazine are dose related—the higher the dose, the more likely the beneficial response. However, higher doses tend to result in various side effects. The most common of these side effects, which occur in approximately 15 to 30 percent of patients, include decreased appetite, headaches (especially in the front part of the head), nausea, and vomiting. Once the patient is in remission, the same dose should be taken for maintenance treatment.

Other 5-ASA Medications

The dose-limiting side effects of sulfasalazine led to the development of sulfa-free 5-ASA medications. Oral preparations include mesalamine (Asacol, Pentasa), balsalazide (Colazal), and olsalazine (Dipentum). The improvement with these medications is similar to that noted with sulfasalazine. Greater improvement with mesalamine is noted with higher doses, which are well tolerated because mesalamine medications do not contain sulfa. Doses can often be increased without an increase in side effects. It is therefore possible to start treatment, or gradually increase treatment, with higher dosages, based on the patient's need.

5-ASA medications also help to sustain remission in patients with mild-to-moderate colitis that results from either Crohn disease or ulcerative colitis. The treatment has minimal side effects. In Crohn disease, treatment with mesalamine may also reduce the risk of disease recurrence among patients who have had surgery to bring their disease under control. Recent data also suggest that mesalamine may decrease the risk of colon cancer in people with ulcerative colitis. No data are available yet regarding risk reduction in patients with Crohn colitis.

Today, many doctors prefer to prescribe mesalamine rather than sulfasalazine, to avoid the potential side effects of the sulfa in sulfasalazine. Mesalamine treatment is safe and well tolerated by children, despite dosages that are higher than those taken by adults (when the amount of medication per weight is compared). Unfortunately, the tablet formulations cannot be broken or chewed, and a pharmacist cannot make liquid preparations without losing the beneficial action of the medication. For children unable to swallow whole tablets or capsules, however, the capsule can be opened, and the granules can be placed in applesauce.

Toxicity of 5-ASA Medications

Symptoms of possible toxicity from sulfasalazine are decreased appetite, headaches (especially in the front part of the head), nausea, and vomiting. Adverse reactions to sulfa can also, on rare occasions, include rash, fever, and other symptoms and signs of severe allergic reaction. Sulfasalazine can reduce the absorption of folic acid from the small intestine into the bloodstream and can therefore cause anemia. To prevent this complication, children should take daily supplemental folic acid while on this medication. Sulfasalazine can cause reversible infertility in males by its effects on sperm. (This problem disappears when the patient stops taking the medication.) Sulfasalazine is safe to take during conception and pregnancy.

The other 5-ASA medications seldom have toxic effects. Kidney toxicity can rarely occur with mesalamine. Commonly obtained lab tests can help monitor for this potential side effect. Mesalamine is safe during conception and pregnancy and has no effect on male fertility. As with all medications, read the information on the 5-ASA drugs provided by the pharmacist and discuss with the health care team any questions you have.

5-ASA Medications in Ulcerative Proctosigmoiditis

Topical (surface medication) 5-ASA preparations are often prescribed for people with inflammation in the lower portions of the large intestine (the rectum and sigmoid colon). Mesalamine suppositories and enemas (brand names Canasa and Rowasa) are associated with higher remission rates and greater clinical improvement than steroid-based topical treatments (see below for information on corticosteroids).

Topical mesalamine treatment is more effective than oral treatment when colitis is restricted to the lowest part of the colon, although combined topical and oral treatment often produces greater improvement than either treatment alone. Once in remission, patients should continue to take not only daily oral treatment, but also topical treatment three to four times each week, to maintain remission.

Corticosteroids

Perhaps the best known of the medications used to induce remission are corticosteroids (CS). Common brand names of CS are Prednisone, Medrol, Pediapred, and Prelone. These drugs can rapidly bring on remission, controlling the most troubling symptoms within days or, at most, weeks. This is especially true with inflammatory symptoms, such as fever and arthritis. Corticosteroids work systemically—that is, throughout the body. Because these medications are effective wherever the inflammation is located in the digestive system, they are useful in treating both Crohn disease and ulcerative colitis. Between 80 and 90 percent of patients achieve a remission with CS treatment. Corticosteroids do not cure IBD, however, and there is no long-term benefit in the continued use of this class of medications.

Corticosteroids are known as much for their adverse side effects as for their positive effects. The side effects of CS increase the longer they are used. The more doses a patient takes, the greater and more serious the side effects. Because of side effects, patients can use these medications for only a limited time. A sudden stop of corticosteroids can also cause dangerous side effects, so patients must follow a schedule for tapering off CS.

Doctors usually prescribe these medications at relatively high doses for a short time to bring on relief of symptoms. Once symptoms are under control, the dose is slowly reduced, and eventually the medication is stopped. Corticosteroids should be used only for induction and not as a maintenance medication. In fact, many experts do not consider a patient to be truly in remission until she is symptom-free and not taking CS.

The side effects associated with the long-term use of CS are displayed in table 10.3. As we have learned more about CS use over the years, recommendations for their use have changed. These changes include

- limiting the accumulated dose of these medications—that is, the total amount a patient takes over time
- careful and timely weaning—CS should not be stopped too quickly or all at once
- combining corticosteroids with immunomodulators to reduce the required dose of CS
- giving newer forms of CS with less severe side effects
- careful monitoring for side effects

Table 10.3. Side effects of corticosteroids

Short-term

• Increased appetite	• Accelerated bone loss (weaker bones)
• Weight gain, especially in the face, upper trunk, and back	• Headache
	• Increased blood pressure
• Stomach irritation	• Night sweats
• Insomnia	• Flushing
• Fluid retention	• Acne

Long-term

• Vulnerability to infections (lowered immunity)	• Drug interactions (discuss with doctor or pharmacist)
• Muscle weakness, especially around the shoulder and hip muscles	• Poor wound healing
	• Stretch marks
• Elevated blood sugar	• Personality changes (irritability, psychosis, depression)
• Bone death (avascular necrosis) of the head of the thigh bone or upper arm bone	• Acne
	• Irregular periods
• Accelerated bone loss (weaker bones)	• Delayed growth
	• Increased facial and body hair
• Cataracts	• Glaucoma
• High blood pressure	• Adrenal gland suppression

For moderate and severe disease, systemic corticosteroids (listed in table 10.4) are given by mouth to a maximum of 40 to 60 milligrams per day (mg/day). This dose may be modified if certain medications, which affect the liver metabolism (breakdown) of corticosteroids, are taken at the same time. Drinking large amounts of grapefruit juice slows the liver's ability to break down corticosteroids, so you need to limit the amount of grapefruit juice your child drinks while taking these medications.

If corticosteroids are first given more than once per day, the dosage may be switched to once in the morning when an improvement is seen. This switch helps decrease some of the short-term side effects of CS. For teenagers, the cosmetic effects of CS (for example, weight gain or acne) are the biggest problems with using these medications.

If oral corticosteroids (those taken by mouth) are not having an effect, or if the patient is hospitalized, CS are generally given intravenously (through an IV) several times during the day. If there is no response within a week or two, it is unlikely that there will be a response to this class of drugs. Patients who do not respond to CS are called *steroid resistant*.

Among patients who are helped by CS, oral steroid treatments continue for several weeks, and then doctors start to gradually decrease the dose. Some patients may be able to discontinue their CS without a flare of their disease, but other patients are classified as *steroid dependent*. That is because they will have a flare when they reduce or stop their CS dose. Because many patients are steroid dependent, corticosteroids are commonly combined with immunomodulators. The com-

Table 10.4. Pill, intravenous, and rectal forms of corticosteroids

Pill (oral)
Prednisone, prednisolone, budesonide

Intravenous
Methylprednisolone (Solu-Medrol), hydrocortisone (Solu-Cortef)

Rectal
Colocort, Cortifoam, budesonide

bination may start as soon as corticosteroids are prescribed or after it becomes clear that a patient is steroid dependent. Steroid-dependent patients require an increase in CS dose to control their symptoms again.

Corticosteroids are powerful medications that must be taken every day, exactly as prescribed. Missing doses, or decreasing the amount of CS too quickly after taking them for several weeks, can have serious and bad effects on the body. The problem occurs because of the natural actions of an organ in the body called the adrenal gland, which produces a natural corticosteroid called cortisone. Cortisone is an important hormone with widespread effects on the workings of cells in the body. The adrenal gland can sense how much cortisone is in the bloodstream and whether it is the natural kind or its manufactured equivalent (such as prednisone). If high levels of corticosteroids are detected, the adrenal gland stops producing any cortisone on its own. Once it senses that the CS levels in the bloodstream are lower, it starts producing cortisone again, very slowly.

If the person is left without any corticosteroids in the bloodstream, many problems can develop (table 10.5). If CS are stopped suddenly, the adrenal gland will not sense the need to resume producing cortisone quickly enough to avoid leaving the body with no cortisone at all. With slow tapering off, the adrenal gland will return to its usual level of functioning without long-term bad effects, because the body will have a supply of cortisone to draw on.

In addition to giving your child corticosteroids every day, exactly as your child's doctor prescribed, it is important to notify the doctor if a child taking CS develops an infection, needs surgery, or is involved in a serious accident. These unusual stresses to the body may require temporary increases in the CS treatment. Normally, the adrenal gland would be pushed to make more cortisone under these stressful conditions. However, it is incapable of doing so when a patient is taking corticosteroids.

Finally, if a patient develops an illness with vomiting and is unable to keep oral corticosteroids in their stomach long enough for the medication to be absorbed, the patient should go to the hospital. Doctors in the hospital will start an IV, and CS will be given through that route.

Table 10.5. Symptoms of stopping corticosteroids too quickly after long-term use

• Nausea with or without vomiting	• Muscle pain
• Fatigue	• Fever
• Loss of appetite	• Joint pains
• Shortness of breath or difficulty in breathing	• Dizziness
• Low blood sugar	• Skin peeling
• Low blood pressure	• Fainting
• Feeling of uneasiness or general discomfort	• Irregular heartbeats

To minimize the side effects of CS use, patients with IBD affecting the rectum and sigmoid colon (lower part of the colon) may be treated with enemas containing hydrocortisone (for example, Cortenema, Cortifoam). Only about 25 percent of the enema dose is absorbed into the bloodstream. Although patients may still experience side effects from the enemas, the side effects might be less severe.

Budesonide (Entocort) is a corticosteroid medication that offers an alternative to systemic corticosteroids for patients with disease involving the last regions of the small bowel and the first part of the colon. This medication has a coating that allows it to bypass the stomach and be released slowly, so that only these two sections of the intestinal tract are targeted. Budesonide is also available as an enema, for patients with disease of the rectum and sigmoid.

Budesonide is a form of steroid that is rapidly broken down in the body after passing through the digestive tract. This rapid breakdown of the drug greatly decreases its side effects. A special form of this medication, given as a pill, releases the active part of the drug in the ileum (the end of the small intestine). The medication stays active in the first part of the large intestine before being broken down. Therefore, this medication is not likely to help people with ulcerative colitis, which involves the lower part of the large intestine. For people with Crohn disease that is limited to the ileum and first part of the colon, budesonide is a potential induction medication. One important aspect of this medication is that the capsule must be swallowed whole to obtain the right effect, so the many children who aren't able to swallow pills cannot take budesonide, and this limits its use in children.

Budesonide is active when it is in contact with the inflamed lining of the intestines, and therefore dosing of this medication is not the same as for systemic corticosteroids. It is not as effective as systemic corticosteroids—the response rate is only about 60 percent. Small amounts of this medication are absorbed across the lining of the intestine, and from there it is carried to the liver, where it is broken down. Patients taking medications that reduce the liver's ability to break down drugs may need to have their budesonide dose adjusted. As with other corticosteroids, large amounts of grapefruit juice increase the bodywide effects of budesonide. Therefore, drinking large amounts of grapefruit juice should be avoided.

Though budesonide causes fewer side effects than other CS, and the side effects are slower to develop, patients are still at risk for them. As with systemic corticosteroids, budesonide doses should decrease slowly, to prevent the development of adrenal gland problems. Also similar to systemic corticosteroids, the use of this medication is to control active symptoms related to IBD, and there is no long-term benefit of taking budesonide in the prevention of disease relapse.

Immunomodulators and Biologics

An immunomodulator is a drug that has an effect on the immune system. A biologic medication is made of a protein (rather than of chemical compounds) and must be given by IV or by injection.

The immunomodulator group of medications (table 10.6) are prescribed to directly affect the autoimmune process in people with inflammatory bowel disease. The most commonly used immunomodulator is 6-mercaptopurine (6-MP; brand name Purinethol). 6-MP and a closely related medication, azathioprine (brand name Imuran) are given by mouth. Formal studies have shown that 6-MP is very effective at maintaining remission in children with Crohn disease. These medications have been used for many years and show good long-term safety. There is also experience using these medications as maintenance treatment in ulcerative colitis. Deciding whether to prescribe an immunomodulator for a child with severe ulcerative colitis is some-times a difficult decision, because surgical removal of the colon (*colec-tomy*) might be a preferable treatment. Discussions between the patient, parents, and health care team are very important in these situations.

Methotrexate is another immunomodulator that can maintain re-mission in Crohn disease. This medication is given once a week as an injection under the skin. Patients who are responding well to metho-trexate may be able to switch to an oral form of this medicine. The drug's effectiveness is well established in adults, and there is already a good experience in children. Doctors usually select methotrexate for patients who do not respond well to 6-MP. It has not been well studied in patients with ulcerative colitis. While methotrexate is generally safe and very well tolerated, it can harm a developing fetus and therefore *should not be used by any women who might become pregnant* while on the medication.

The use of immunomodulating drugs in the treatment of IBD has greatly improved the likelihood of response, while allowing reduction or discontinuation of corticosteroid medications in children. As stud-ies continue to confirm the long-term safety of these medications, doc-tors who treat children and adolescents have become increasingly willing to use these drugs more frequently and for longer duration. Most of the drugs used to treat IBD, including the widely used 5-ami-nosalicylates and corticosteroids, have an effect on immune system actions. In this section we review the role of other immunomodulating medications in the treatment of children and teens with IBD.

Table 10.6. Immunomodulators

Azathioprine (Imuran)
6-Mercaptopurine (Purinethol)
Methotrexate
Cyclosporine (Neoral)
Tacrolimus (Prograf)

Only experienced gastroenterologists should prescribe immunomodulating and biologic agents.

Reasons for Choosing Immunomodulating Drugs in Children

While corticosteroids are effective in reducing disease activity in many children with acute ulcerative colitis or Crohn disease, there are clear reasons for adding immunosuppressive medications:

- Some patients do not respond to corticosteroid treatments.
- The potential side effects of corticosteroids (discussed above), especially long term, are severe.

Azathioprine and 6-Mercaptopurine

Azathioprine (AZA) and 6-MP are currently among the best studied of the steroid-sparing drugs used to treat IBD in children and teens. Many pediatric gastroenterologists include this class of drugs (6-MP, AZA) in the initial treatment of children with newly diagnosed, moderate-to-severe Crohn disease. In ulcerative colitis, these medications have been shown to increase corticosteroid-free periods, decrease frequency of relapses, and improve gains in height and weight in children and adolescents.

Some children who receive these drugs are unable to continue treatment because of either a serious reaction to the medication (such as pancreatitis or fever) or intolerance (nausea, abdominal pain, or repeat infections). These drugs can also suppress production of cells in the bone marrow, causing the white blood cells to decrease, and can cause inflammation of the liver. AZA and 6-MP may also slightly increase a person's risk of developing a cancer in the future. Patients should not receive live-virus vaccines while taking these drugs. It is important to seek medical attention if the patient develops high fever, is exposed to chicken pox (if the child has not been previously infected with this virus), or shows other signs and symptoms of potentially serious infectious illnesses.

At least 87 percent of patients who can take AZA or 6-MP are able to decrease dosage or discontinue corticosteroid treatment. AZA and 6-MP are important drugs in maintaining reduced disease activity, or remission, in patients with severe disease whose remission was achieved with cyclosporine or tacrolimus (see below). Under these circumstances, AZA and 6-MP may lengthen remission in ulcerative colitis and Crohn disease, which may delay the time to colectomy.

Deciding on the best dose of AZA or 6-MP in individual patients is an area of active study. Measuring blood levels of a breakdown product of 6-MP, called 6-thioguanine (6-TG), the active ingredient of the drug, may lead to improved treatment in some patients with lingering disease activity. Furthermore, metabolites, which increase the risk of hepatic (liver) side effects, can be monitored and the dosage adjusted or the drug discontinued if necessary.

Methotrexate

Approximately 18 percent of children cannot tolerate AZA or 6-MP. For these patients, as well as for those who are also corticosteroid dependent, additional drug choices are necessary. Based largely on the results of adult studies, pediatric gastroenterologists may use methotrexate (MTX) in such patients. Much of the information about the safety of MTX in children comes from extensive long-term experience in children with juvenile rheumatoid arthritis (JRA) who receive MTX.

The possible development of liver scarring (fibrosis or cirrhosis) is a concern with the use of MTX. Studies directly addressed this issue in children who received long-term MTX for JRA, however, and the risk of liver scarring appears to be rare.

In contrast to its use in JRA, MTX in IBD is usually given by injection rather than by mouth, to reduce the likelihood of digestive side effects. Safety monitoring is essential with MTX and includes regular reviews of the complete blood count and liver enzyme tests. A child with acute or chronic liver disease (with the exception of primary sclerosing cholangitis [PSC]) should not receive MTX. In addition, children with chronic lung disease should have a lung function test and consultation with a lung specialist if they are to receive MTX, because of the potential risk of serious reactions in the lung. This complication was not seen in lung function tests performed in children with JRA who were treated with long-term MTX.

Cyclosporine-A and Tacrolimus

Use of cyclosporine-A or tacrolimus (FK506) should be considered only in patients with severe cases of ulcerative colitis or Crohn disease that do not respond to traditional medications. Both medications are strong immune suppressors—that is, they severely lower a person's immunity. It is still uncertain whether the harsh potential side effects of these medications outweigh their benefits.

Cyclosporine-A

Several small studies in adults found a possible short-term benefit to intravenous cyclosporine-A treatment for patients with severe ulcerative colitis (disease that did not respond to other treatments). With or without the addition of steroids, cyclosporine-A treatment decreased the need for emergency removal of the colon (colectomy). When treatment with this drug stops, though, the relapse rate is very high. If cyclosporine is to be used, it should be prescribed with the understanding that colectomy most likely will still be necessary within a year.

No studies have evaluated cyclosporine-A in children with severe Crohn disease. Studies in adults have shown that low-dose cyclosporine-A does not bring or maintain remission in patients with long-term, active Crohn disease. High-dose cyclosporine-A may help achieve remission, but it is associated with serious and harmful effects.

Cyclosporine-A can cause toxicity to the kidneys, high blood pressure, nervous-system side effects, and nausea and vomiting. Swelling of the gums and increased hair growth usually happen only with cyclosporine-A. *Pneumocystis jiroveci* pneumonia (formerly known as *Pneumocystis carinii* pneumonia), an unusual infection seen only in immunosuppressed individuals, may develop during cyclosporine-A treatment. Therefore, doctors normally prescribe treatment with antibiotics against *P. jiroveci* when treating patients with cyclosporine-A.

Post-transplant lymphoproliferative disease (infrequently complicated by lymphoma) is a rare complication of cyclosporine treatments and is reported primarily in patients who have undergone solid organ transplants.

Tacrolimus (FK506)

Tacrolimus, which is taken only by mouth, is a stronger immuno-suppressive medication than cyclosporine-A. It is also more reliably absorbed from the intestine into the bloodstream. In the only study of tacrolimus treatment in children, nine of fourteen children with ste-roid-resistant severe colitis achieved short-term remission. This study included children with ulcerative colitis and Crohn colitis. No long-term data on these patients are available.

Similar to cyclosporine-A, tacrolimus can cause kidney toxicity, high blood pressure, nervous-system side effects, and nausea and vom-iting, and can increase the risk of acquiring *P. jiroveci* pneumonia. As with cyclosporine-A, doctors normally prescribe treatment with anti-biotics against *P. jiroveci* when treating patients with tacrolimus. Post-transplant lymphoproliferative disease (infrequently complicated by lymphoma) is a rare complication of tacrolimus treatments and is re-ported primarily in patients who have undergone solid organ trans-plants.

Antitumor Necrosis Factor-α Antibody

The antitumor necrosis factor-α (alpha) antibody (anti-TNF-α) class of *biologic medications* (see "New Treatments in Trials in Adults," below) has greatly influenced the course of illness in many children and ado-lescents with difficult-to-control IBD. Reported benefits include

- disease remission
- healing of fistulas
- reduction and end of corticosteroid treatments
- improved growth in patients who respond

Infliximab (brand name Remicade) is a manufactured antibody that interferes with the inflammatory process in Crohn disease and ulcer-ative colitis. This medication can be extremely effective in bringing both diseases into quick, steroid-free remission. It is a systemic medi-cation, given intravenously. Infliximab will take effect wherever the inflammation is located. Since the drug can have a dramatic response, doctors use it for patients with very active Crohn disease or ulcerative colitis, including those who are not responding to corticosteroids.

A significant number of children who receive infliximab will improve with this treatment, even if they have not responded to prior therapies. In one of the largest studies conducted in children with Crohn disease (the REACH study performed by Dr. Hyams and colleagues), 112 children with active Crohn disease were treated with three doses of infliximab. The second dose was given two weeks after the first dose, and the third dose was given six weeks after the first dose. Ten weeks after the first dose, 88 percent of children had improved. They were then assigned to receive the medication either every two months or every three months. The group treated every two months was more likely to stay in remission then the every-three-month group. Because of the results of this study, the recommended treatment plan for a child receiving infliximab is to receive three doses in the first six weeks, then a scheduled dose every two months. Depending on how effective the medication is, your child's physician may choose to vary the dose or interval. Response to this medication is fairly prompt, though, and if your child does not respond in the first three to six months, other treatments may need to be considered.

Side effects may be acute (occurring during or within a few hours after the infusion), or delayed (up to seven days after the infusion). Shortness of breath or rash can occur in a small percentage of children

Rare postmarketing cases of an aggressive lymphoma have been reported in adolescents and young adult patients with Crohn disease treated with Remicade. This rare type of T cell lymphoma has a very aggressive disease course and is usually fatal. All hepatosplenic T cell lymphomas associated with Remicade have occurred in patients on concomitant treatment with azathioprine or 6-mercaptopurine.

during the infusion, but these side effects require no treatment. More severe acute reactions include anaphylaxis, in which the above reactions are accompanied by a fall in blood pressure, sometimes with extensive redness or hives over the body. Delayed reactions include fever, joint pains or joint swelling (arthritis), headache, and malaise (general ill feeling). Rare, serious complications on anti-TNF-α therapy have been reported. These include increased susceptibility to tuberculosis, invasive fungal infections, and herpetic skin infections. In addition, patients on long-term anti-TNF therapy are at increased risk of developing lymphoma. Fortunately, these serious complications are very rare. Newer anti-TNF-α preparations are being studied. A completely humanized form, adalimumab (Humira), which is effective in patients with reactions to infliximab, was recently approved for the treatment of Crohn disease in adults.

There is evidence that infliximab can have a beneficial effect in some patients with ulcerative colitis whose disease is not responding to other medications. However, patients with UC who respond to infliximab are at risk of a colitis relapse as well as the side effects of the infliximab. Therefore, the UC patient should be aware of surgery as an alternative to long-term immunosuppression.

Infliximab is well studied and approved for use in adults and children with Crohn disease. Since this is still a relatively new medication, major questions about its use remain. Most important, long-term side effects are still unknown, although a black box warning was recently added for Remicade. Treatment with anti-TNF medications carries with it higher risks of cancer and infections. Patients receiving anti-TNF medications should not receive live vaccines.

Other Antitumor Necrosis Factor Antibodies

The dramatic success of infliximab in treating children with Crohn disease whose disease had been unresponsive to other medications has led to the development of two other medications similar to infliximab. These medications are adalimumab (Humira) and certolizumab

(Cimzia). Like the other anti-TNF-α medications, both of these medications are also proteins that block the action of the inflammatory chemical tumor necrosis factor alpha, and both have been shown highly effective in treating Crohn disease in adults. The main difference between these medications and infliximab is how they are given: while infliximab is given as an intravenous infusion (going into the vein) every two months, adalimumab and certolizumab are given as injections under the skin (shots) every two to four weeks. Although we have less experience with these newer TNF inhibitors than with infliximab, they can be useful in children who either have not responded to infliximab or have developed an allergic reaction to infliximab. Treatment trials of these agents and newer therapies are discussed in the section below, on new treatments.

Antibiotics

Antibiotics play a role in the treatment of inflammatory bowel disease. Doctors often prescribe them for mild flares and for specific symptoms, including *perianal* complications (complications around the anus) from Crohn disease. Sometimes doctors prescribe antibiotics in addition to the other medications listed above to help bring flares under control.

Patients with IBD have a problem with the way their own immune system works. Normally, the immune system provides protection from invading bacteria and in this way prevents infections. In IBD, although no identifiable infection is present, the immune system acts as if it were responding to invading bacteria, attacking areas of the bowel as if an infection were present.

A great deal of research has focused on understanding this disturbance in the immune system. Research shows that bacteria that normally live in the intestine play a role in this process. Normally, there is a balance between these bacteria and immune system activity. A loss of this balance in IBD may result in chronic inflammation. Therefore, while no identifiable bacteria cause IBD, antibiotics can help reduce the inflammation by changing the amount and type of bacteria that are in the intestine.

Antibiotics have more effect in Crohn disease than ulcerative colitis. This may be partly because ulcerative colitis affects only the lining of the bowel, whereas Crohn disease affects the lining and deeper wall of the bowel. Therefore, bacteria can get deeper into the intestines in Crohn disease and cause complications such as fistulas. Fistulas are abnormal, inflammatory openings from a portion of the intestine to other nearby structures, including skin, bladder, and vagina. Treatment with antibiotics against the bacteria that normally live in the bowel helps heal fistulas. In addition, antibiotics help Crohn disease patients who have disease activity in their colon and around their anus.

Metronidazole (brand name Flagyl) and ciprofloxacin (brand name Cipro) are the two most studied antibiotics in Crohn disease. Because of potential side effects of these drugs, neither can be used long term, but a course of several weeks of one or both of these antibiotics can be useful for some patients. Clarithromycin (brand name Biaxin) is an antibiotic frequently used for common childhood infections, and it has been used effectively in pediatric Crohn disease. Another antibiotic, rifaximin (brand name Xifaxin), has also been helpful in adults and children with Crohn disease.

Although no specific bacteria or infections are known to cause IBD, *Clostridium difficile* is one particular bacterium that deserves special mention. *C. difficile* (often called *C. diff* by doctors) is a bacterium that can grow in the bowel after a patient has been exposed to antibiotics for any reason. It can cause a bowel inflammation resembling the colitis of IBD and has been associated with disease flares in people with IBD. Even though this infection is *caused* by exposure to antibiotics, *C. diff* can be treated effectively with an antibiotic, metronidazole, and people with IBD flares may take this antibiotic to treat *C. difficile*.

In ulcerative colitis, the treatment of a severe flare may include antibiotics because the damaged bowel lining may become infected as a result of the damage from the disease process and the presence of bacteria in the colon. If C. *difficile* is found in someone with ulcerative colitis, this infection should be treated with antibiotics.

Probiotics

A different type of treatment that works directly on the inflamed lining of the intestines is probiotic therapy. Probiotics are live, noninfectious bacteria ("good bacteria," similar to those found in yogurt and other foods). In theory, these bacteria improve the protective mechanisms of the bowel and alter intestinal inflammation caused by an immune response. Certain types of probiotic bacteria have been shown in animal studies to improve inflammation, but more studies are needed in humans. Studies have shown that probiotics can lessen or prevent a complication of colon surgery called *pouchitis*. Some strains of these bacteria are naturally resistant to stomach acids and bile and are available in foods such as yogurt. They are also available commercially as powders of live bacteria that a person can add to foods. Some other types of probiotics that are more sensitive to stomach acid are becoming commercially available in coated microsphere formulations, which work similarly to the coated 5-ASA preparations described above. These coated preparations are able to bypass the harsh stomach acid, releasing the probiotic bacteria downstream in the intestine. Once released, the bacteria change the workings of the digestive tract immune cells, nonimmune cells, and "bad" bacteria that cause inflammation. Medical studies have not clearly demonstrated a benefit of probiotics in the treatment of Crohn disease or ulcerative colitis. However, research to see if they are useful continues.

Summary of Induction and Remission Treatment

New treatments for children and teens with IBD continue to be developed, providing additional options for patients with nonresponsive disease, often leading to reduced use of or stopping of corticosteroid medications. As new medications become available, special considerations in children, such as bone abnormalities, growth, infection risks, and differences in drug breakdown, will need to be studied.

For induction of remission in children and adolescents with mild to moderately active ulcerative colitis, doctors usually recommend 5-aminosalicylates. For children and adolescents with a greater level of UC activity, doctors use corticosteroids.

For patients with Crohn disease, doctors use combinations of medications. Antibiotics with or without 5-aminosalicylates can be tried if there is mild disease activity. Crohn disease that is more active is treated with corticosteroids, budesonide, or even infliximab.

Once inflammatory bowel disease is under control, treatment turns to a maintenance program. For maintenance therapy, the 5-aminosalicylates are the mainstay of treatment in people with mild to moderate ulcerative colitis. For people with ulcerative colitis who continue to relapse (have flares), surgical removal of the colon (colectomy) or immunomodulator treatment is an option.

With mild Crohn disease, 5-aminosalicylates have sometimes been used for maintenance treatment. For people with Crohn disease who continue to relapse and show moderately or severely active Crohn disease, immunomodulator treatment or anti-TNF therapy is an option.

Nutritional Therapy

The role of nutrition as supplemental therapy for growth and sexual development is discussed in greater detail in chapter 13. In this chapter we discuss nutrition as a primary therapy to induce remission in patients with Crohn disease. Studies have shown that nutritional supplements can be as effective as corticosteroids in inducing remission.

In nutritional therapy, specialized formulas are used to make sure that patients are receiving all the nutrients, vitamins and minerals, they need for healing and growth. The formulas can be taken orally, but because they are often not palatable, they are administered through tube. A tube (nasogastric, or NG, tube) is passed through the child's nose into the stomach to administer the formula. During the treatment period, which in most cases is six to eight weeks, this may be the primary food that your child will receive. When the child is in remission, the tube feeds are decreased and normal food is reintroduced.

Although NG feeds are effective in inducing remission, patients treated with this method are more likely to flare when the feedings are stopped.

New Treatments in Trials in Adults

Since the groundbreaking work showing the usefulness of infliximab in Crohn disease, a large number of new potential treatments have entered into clinical trials for both Crohn disease and ulcerative colitis. It is most common for clinical trials to be done first in adults, and then in children. In some cases, clinical trials in children take place at the same time as trials in adults. It is worth noting that the first patient ever treated with infliximab was a child.

The newer treatments beyond infliximab have continued to build on the success of this biologic medication. Biologic treatments are made of a protein, instead of a chemical compound. They are easy to translate from a scientific observation in the laboratory into a new treatment. However, major disadvantages of biologics are the cost and inconvenience—they must be given by IV or injection. Most proteins are not easily digested when taken by mouth and would therefore be ineffective if given this way.

Infliximab is the first generation of anti-TNF biologic medications. Tumor necrosis factor (TNF) is a protein found in the body that is strongly involved in the inflammation caused by Crohn disease. Infliximab is an antibody that binds very specifically to TNF and helps clear it from the body, thereby decreasing inflammation in Crohn disease and ulcerative colitis.

A potential disadvantage of infliximab is that 25 percent of this protein consists of a mouse protein. With repeated treatments, the immune system may begin to recognize this foreign protein and develop antibodies against the drug, which decreases its effectiveness and increases its side effects. The manufacturers of second-generation anti-TNF biologics have been trying to make more humanlike proteins that may avoid this disadvantage. The completely humanized anti-TNF Humira, which is already approved for treating rheumatoid arthritis in the United States, has recently been approved for adult treatment of Crohn disease. In a study of 172 adults receiving 40 mg of Humira every other week for treatment of CD, 36 percent were still in remission after fifty-six weeks. A third anti-TNF inhibitor, certolizumab (Cimzia), has also been FDA approved for adults with Crohn disease and has comparable effectiveness to Remicade and Humira.

Another promising class of medications is the *selective adhesion molecule inhibitors*. This new class of medications works by an entirely different mechanism than that of the anti-TNF medications. Selective adhesion molecule inhibitors interfere with the ability of white blood cells to enter into the intestinal tissue. (The white cells are the cells mainly involved in the inflammation caused by IBD.) Interrupting this process may reduce the inflammation and improve symptoms of the disease. The first demonstration that this type of approach could be effective was with the drug natalizumab. This humanized antibody binds to a white blood cell protein called alpha-4 integrin. This medication has now been approved by the FDA to treat resistant Crohn disease in adults. A small pediatric study suggests that this drug may help children. One concern about natalizumab, however, is that it appears to increase the risk of developing progressive multifocal leukoencephalopathy, a rare infection of the central nervous system.

One recent study suggested that the cellular growth factor GM-CSF (sargramostim) was found to be effective in inducing remission in adults with Crohn disease. The researchers who proposed this type of treatment believe that this drug works by increasing the activity of neutrophils. (Neutrophils are a type of white blood cell that is critical for the body's immediate defense response against infections.) Additional studies will be necessary to find out whether this medication will be effective in larger numbers of patients.

Severe ulcerative colitis remains a difficult problem. While hospitalized patients who fail to respond to steroids often do respond to cyclosporine, this drug has considerable possible toxicity. An alternative treatment may be the biologic medication visilizumab. This medication works by destroying activated T cells. T cells are critical to the forceful immune response that occurs in the colon in ulcerative colitis. The number of activated T cells temporarily drops after treatment with visilizumab. Early studies are very promising in turning around even severe and difficult cases of ulcerative colitis. Additional, more thorough, studies are needed before the drug will be considered for approval.

An intriguing new treatment is the use of intentional infection with non-disease-causing worm eggs. The type of worms used (*Trichuris suis*) are microscopic and normally found in hogs. They do not cause disease and do not make a permanent home in people. The theory is that intestinal infection with worms reprograms the immune system. Such reprogramming reduces the abnormal immune response that causes CD and UC. Worm infestations in humans were common until very recent times, when hygiene became widespread. Early studies have been promising, but many additional studies are needed before worm treatment will become a useful treatment in adults or children.

Many other investigational treatments are in earlier phases of exploration. This is an exciting time, filled with promise for better treatment of patients with Crohn disease and those with ulcerative colitis.

Therapy for Crohn disease and ulcerative colitis is changing rapidly, and it can be challenging for a family to weigh the risks and benefits of various treatments. Patients and families should ask as many questions as necessary to become comfortable with the treatment of IBD. In response, health care professionals should provide information in clear language. Teaching materials such as pamphlets, books, and articles, and contact with support groups, are often very helpful. In this day of searching online for information, each family should be encouraged to get as much information as possible from their health care team, rather than from the Internet. Online information often does not relate to children and is not always accurate. You can rely on information from the major IBD foundations and associations (such as the Crohn's and Colitis Foundation of America), and from the Centers for Disease Control and Prevention (the CDC) and the National Institutes of Health (the NIH), but again, information about disease and treatment in adults may not be applicable in children.

❦ 11
Surgery

Surgery is an important part of the treatment for both Crohn disease and ulcerative colitis. Surgery is not necessarily a last resort with IBD as it is with other conditions. In fact, doctors often recommend early surgical treatment along with medications, and a large number of patients with IBD will require some type of surgery during the course of their illness. For some people, surgery may be used early in the treatment of their disease.

Who Needs Surgery?

Although deciding whether to perform surgery for IBD often carries with it a great deal of worry, in certain situations, the decision to operate is made relatively easily. These situations include cases of uncontrollable bleeding, perforations (holes in the intestine), obstruction (complete blockage), and intestinal cancer. In such *emergent* (urgent) situations, the type of intestinal disease (Crohn disease or ulcerative colitis) is not an important consideration, because surgery is the only helpful approach to treatment. When surgery is to be performed *electively* (by choice), however, the decision to undergo an operation, and deciding when it should be performed, is more difficult.

The goals of IBD treatment are

to ease or stop symptoms,
to improve general health, and
to improve growth, sexual development, and dietary condition.

The purpose of surgery is to reach these goals when medication treatment has failed or become too toxic, while trying to save as much of the intestine as possible. The decision about whether surgery is necessary is made based on medical history, x-ray tests (chapter 8), and endoscopic exams (chapter 9).

Patients and their families should discuss surgery, including the potential advantages and disadvantages, with the entire medical team, which usually includes many specialists, such as a pediatric gastroenterologist, an IBD surgeon, a nurse practitioner, a nutritionist, and a psychologist. All treatment options should be discussed thoroughly. Only in this way can everyone feel confident that the best decision is being made about the next step in treatment.

In terms of choosing a surgeon, keep in mind that it is important for the surgeon to be familiar with the special features of caring for children and adolescents with IBD. The surgeon should also be familiar with different surgical techniques, including state-of-the-art advances in the field of IBD surgery.

Support organizations can provide essential information on quality of life after surgery. It might also be helpful for children who are facing surgery to talk to other children who had similar operations done. In addition, it is always preferable to make home care arrangements, and take care of health insurance issues, ahead of time.

General Terms

Two main techniques are used to perform IBD surgery: laparotomy and laparoscopy. *Laparotomy,* or open surgery, is the method requiring only one abdominal incision (cut), but it is a somewhat larger cut. A more recently developed method, called *laparoscopy,* makes use of instruments that are inserted into the abdomen through several small openings. Laparoscopy leaves several very small scars.

Laparoscopic surgery may be somewhat more difficult to do and should be done only by a surgeon familiar with the technique. If done by the right surgeon, laparoscopy allows for an easier and faster recovery. At the time of the surgery, though, the surgeon must make the final decision about which type of procedure to use. Sometimes it is necessary to change procedures in the operating room, even when a different surgical procedure was planned.

The types of surgical procedures vary depending on the type of IBD and the reason for surgery. In this chapter, we first review the reasons for surgery and the procedures used for ulcerative colitis. We will then describe the different surgical treatments for Crohn disease.

Surgery for Ulcerative Colitis

Table 11.1 lists the most common reasons for having urgent surgery and for considering surgery for ulcerative colitis. The goal of surgical treatment for ulcerative colitis is to cure the disease. Such surgery involves removing the large intestine, however, and is not undertaken lightly. The surgery can cause complications, and it usually requires lifestyle changes. The type of surgery done depends on the reasons for the operation. Each surgery should be customized for the patient, depending on medical history and test results.

Before describing the surgical procedures for ulcerative colitis, we need to briefly review stomas, appliances, and their care.

The word *stoma* originates from the Greek word for mouth. A surgeon creates a stoma by bringing the intestine out through the skin to the abdominal (belly) wall. The stoma opens to the outside of the

---

Table 11.1. Reasons for surgery to treat ulcerative colitis

Urgent

- uncontrolled bleeding
- a hole in the intestine (perforation)
- intestinal obstruction (blockage)
- extreme swelling of the colon (toxic megacolon)
- cancer of the large intestine (colon cancer)

Optional

- poor response to medication

---

body. The name of the stoma depends on which part of the intestine connects to the skin. For example, the stoma is a *colostomy* if part of the colon (large intestine) was brought out to the skin; an *ileostomy* means the ileum, or second half of the small intestine, is brought out, and so on. There are several types of stomas, such as Kock pouch and Brooke ileostomy, among others.

In the most common type of stoma, called a Brooke ileostomy or colostomy, the end of a loop of intestine is brought out through an opening in the abdomen, folded on itself to form a stoma, and sutured to the skin. The opening is approximately the size of a quarter and the intestine's contents, which are usually pasty in consistency, collect into an *appliance* (a bag that is attached to the skin with adhesive). The bag must be emptied several times a day and changed every few days (figure 11.1).

Most patients (95%) are able to lead normal lives with a stoma, including attending school regularly, participating in sports, and taking part in most normal activities of daily life. The site of the stoma has to be chosen carefully so that it is located on a flat skin surface away from creases, bony areas, and previous scars. The preferred site will

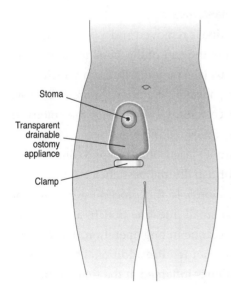

Stoma

Transparent
drainable
ostomy
appliance

Clamp

Figure 11.1. An ostomy appliance. Patients who undergo removal of the colon (because of IBD-related colitis) may require a temporary or permanent ostomy. An external ileostomy allows intestinal contents to empty into a small, discreet plastic sack that can be periodically emptied into a toilet.

locate the bag in an area where intestinal movements can easily drain into it and where emptying the bag is easy. The stoma must be positioned so that clothes fit well, sitting is comfortable, and, when possible, the bag is concealed.

An enterostomal specialist is an important member of the surgical team. He can provide advice about the appropriate type of stoma appliance and can work with the patient to troubleshoot any complications that occur (infection, leakage, and so on).

Types of Surgical Procedures for Ulcerative Colitis

Proctocolectomy with End-Ileostomy

In this procedure the entire large intestine is removed, and the end of the small intestine is brought out as a stoma. This is the least popular type of surgery since it requires a permanent appliance on the abdomen. This procedure is rarely performed now in patients with ulcerative colitis, especially not in children and adolescents. Occasionally, however, this surgery is necessary if the procedure called total colectomy and ileal pouch anal anastomosis has failed.

Total Colectomy with Ileoanal Anastomosis

In this surgery, the large intestine is removed and a pelvic "pouch" (internal reservoir) is created from the end of the small intestine. The reservoir is connected to the anus (the opening through which stool comes out of the body), allowing normal defecation (figure 11.2). This is the most popular choice for colectomy (removal of the colon) to treat ulcerative colitis. It can be performed in several ways.

One-stage operation is the surgery used only in approximately 10 percent of patients, and it is not usually the best choice for patients with IBD (except in special situations). In this procedure, removal of the large intestine, creation of a small intestine pouch, and connection of the pouch to the anus are done in one operation. The advantage of this method is that it does not require additional surgeries or a temporary stoma. If the intestine is inflamed at the time of this op-

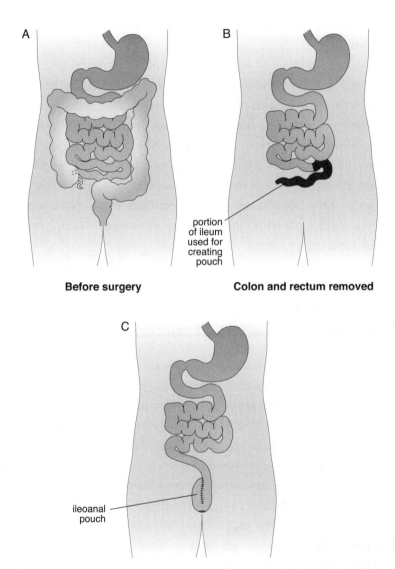

Before surgery   **Colon and rectum removed**

portion
of ileum
used for
creating
pouch

ileoanal
pouch

Figure 11.2. Colectomy with ileoanal pouch. Most patients with ulcerative colitis who undergo colon removal do not require a permanent ileostomy. Instead, a temporary ostomy is created. In subsequent procedures, a portion of the ileum (B) is folded back on itself and pulled down to the anal region (C). Assuming this "J pouch" (ileoanal pouch) can be successfully created, the ileostomy can be closed and a patient can empty intestinal contents through the anus.

eration, however, there is a risk for poor healing, which can lead to problems.

Two-stage operation is a procedure involving removal of the large intestine, creation of the small intestine pouch, and connection to the anus. A temporary stoma on the abdomen is created and kept in place for a few months. The temporary stoma disconnects movement of feces from the intestine to the anus, so no stool passes through the anus. The stoma allows the internal pouch to heal well before stool passes through it. After two or three months, the stoma is closed and the ends of the intestine are reconnected. Once the intestine is reconnected, stool passes through the anus in normal fashion, and the stoma is no longer needed.

The three-stage operation involves first removing the colon and performing the ileostomy (opening in the abdomen). Later, after the patient recovers, the small intestine pouch is formed in a second operation, but the ileostomy remains. Finally, after more time for complete healing, the ileostomy is removed and the intestine is connected to the anus. Three-stage procedures are used when a patient has major intestinal inflammation at the time of the surgery.

After complete recovery from a total colectomy with ileal pouch and anastomosis, regardless of the number of stages, a person usually has an average of four to eight bowel movements a day. To decrease the frequency of bowel movements, patients often receive treatments to train the small intestine pouch to store liquid stool. Additional dietary fiber and medications can also help in decreasing the number of bowel movements. The medications slow the movement of waste through the intestine.

The pouch frequently becomes inflamed (a condition known as *pouchitis*) at some point after the surgery, usually within the first year. Pouchitis attacks can occur a few times each year, but the frequency of attacks usually decreases as time passes. Eventually, pouchitis may stop completely or occur only now and then. Chronic pouchitis that does not go away occurs in only a small number of patients.

Other complications after surgery include pouch leaks, fistula formation (an abnormal opening between the pouch and nearby organs), incontinence (not making it to the bathroom in time), and obstruction (blockage). Blockage happens due to a narrowing at the site where the pouch connects to the anus.

After surgery about 4 percent of patients who had apparent ulcerative colitis turn out to have Crohn disease, despite all the early evidence of ulcerative colitis. These patients tend to have more complications after surgery. In a small number of patients (about 10 percent), the ileal pouch may need to be removed and the ileostomy re-created.

Total Colectomy with Ileorectal Anastomosis

In this type of surgery, most of the large intestine is removed, and a straight connection is made between the end of the small intestine and the rectum (the lowermost part of the large intestine), without creating a pelvic pouch. This procedure is rarely used, since a part of the diseased large intestine is left behind after surgery. Some people believe that quality of life may be somewhat better with this procedure than after a pouch operation, because patients can have fewer bowel movements. However, the risk of ongoing inflammation, and the possible development of cancer in the remaining segment of the large intestine, makes this procedure less desirable. This type of surgery can lead to decreased fertility (difficulties in becoming pregnant) in females, so issues of fertility should be thoroughly discussed beforehand if this is a concern.

Surgery for Crohn Disease

The most common reasons for having surgery, whether urgently or electively, to treat Crohn disease are summarized in table 11.2. Choosing to have elective surgery can be particularly difficult for patients with Crohn disease. In ulcerative colitis, surgery cures the disease. But surgery for Crohn disease does not cure the illness. In fact, there is a real chance that the disease will return at some point after surgery and that the person might need more operations. Nevertheless, elective surgery is still the correct decision for a child with Crohn disease in several situations, as described below. Each case is followed by a description of the most appropriate surgery in these circumstances.

Table 11.2. Reasons for surgery to treat Crohn disease

Urgent

- uncontrolled bleeding
- obstruction (blockage)
- perforation (hole)
- abscess (infections) or fistulizing disease (when Crohn disease causes abnormal openings between organs)

Optional

- failure of medication treatment
    stricture (narrowing in the intestine)
    perianal disease (swelling and sores around the anus)

Scenario 1

A 15-year-old girl has had Crohn disease for three years. Tests showed that the disease is most severe in the last portion of the small intestine. At first, the disease disappeared after steroid treatment, but every time the treatment stopped, the symptoms returned. Her symptoms are usually abdominal pain and bloating, sometimes with diarrhea. The symptoms are often worst after eating, and to avoid symptoms, the child has started to limit the amount that she eats. As a result, this child has become malnourished—her body is not getting the food it needs to grow and stay healthy and strong.

Treatment with medicine that makes the immune system less active was not effective in allowing her to stop steroid treatments and remain well. As a result, she now needs regular intravenous infusions of infliximab. (Infliximab is medicine that suppresses the immune system and works to reduce or prevent inflammation. See chapter 10.) After a year of treatments with infliximab, the symptoms are coming back, and the child is beginning to lose weight again. Follow-up tests show the same localized area of inflammation with some narrowing of the intestine. The child is underweight and short for her age and is just starting to show signs of puberty now.

Why Surgery Might Be Right for This Child

Several factors might make surgery the right choice for this child. First, the child's disease has been resistant to treatment with several different medicines. Although steroids can control some of the symptoms, research shows that steroids are very unlikely to bring on healing. Furthermore, steroids have many negative side effects that become more and more undesirable the longer they are used.

A second point in favor of surgery is that the disease appears to be located in one particular area of the small intestine. This makes it unlikely that a large portion of the intestine will need to be removed.

Finally, it is very important that the child is just about to enter puberty. Puberty in this adolescent girl is already somewhat delayed at this point, and if she has continued active disease throughout this important time of growth and development, she may have permanent growth problems.

Intestinal surgery for Crohn disease in children generally involves removing the least amount of intestine possible, but enough to take care of the intestine that is clearly diseased (figure 11.3). This operation can be performed as a traditional "open" procedure, where a single cut is made in the abdominal wall, followed by examination of the intestine and removal of the diseased segment(s). The surgery can also be done as a laparoscopic procedure, where the intestine is removed using small tools inserted into the abdomen through several small punctures. Laparoscopic surgery for Crohn disease is used more and more often because recovery is faster and there is less pain after surgery. In complicated cases, though, it may be safer to perform the surgery open.

Scenario 2

A 12-year-old child has had Crohn disease for five years. He was treated with steroids after diagnosis. Steroids were not needed again after the first course. The child took mesalamine (an anti-inflammatory) for a few years but stopped using it because he had no symptoms. He remained symptom-free until the past six months, when his family began to notice some bloating after meals. Lately, the bloating has become more uncomfortable, and occasionally the boy vomits after a meal. A few weeks ago, the child suffered from severe pain and vomiting after a meal and was checked by his GI doctor. A very nar-

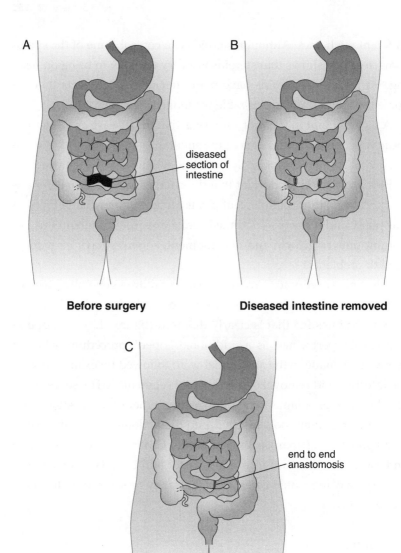

Before surgery

diseased section of intestine

Diseased intestine removed

Healthy sections reconnected

end to end anastomosis

Figure 11.3. Bowel resection and end-to-end anastomosis. In Crohn disease, a small region of bowel sometimes needs to be removed because of inflammation, perforation, or narrowing. In most cases, the diseased section is removed, and the two healthy sections can be reconnected. Assuming the amount of bowel removed is small, intestinal function is usually normal.

rowed part of the ileum was seen on a special x-ray called a barium upper GI study (see chapter 8). The area of intestine before this narrowed part was dilated (enlarged), meaning the intestine above it had begun to stretch out due to the narrowing downstream. A colonoscopy (see chapter 9) was done, and this test showed a normal-looking colon. A course of steroids was given, and the barium x-ray was repeated, but there was no real change in the appearance of the narrowed area, and the symptoms stayed the same.

Why Surgery Might Be Right for This Child

There are a few reasons to believe that treatment with medication will not work for this child. The fact that the intestine is dilated above the narrowing means that the narrowing has been developing over a long time. The lack of change in the appearance of the intestine, even while the child was on steroid therapy, shows that the narrowing may have become fixed like a scar (rather than being due just to inflamed tissue). As a result, surgical treatment called *strictureplasty* may be a good option.

Strictureplasty widens the narrowed intestine to allow easier passage of intestinal contents, although it makes the intestines slightly shorter. The advantage of this type of operation is that the narrowing can be treated without removing a portion of the intestine. In addition, recovery may be faster than it would be if part of the intestine were removed.

Problems with this type of operation include the possibility of the stricture returning, and the possibility of fistula formation at the surgical site.

Scenario 3

A 10-year-old child has had recurrent abscesses (infections) around the anus for years. Finally, the child was diagnosed with Crohn disease and a severe stricture in the rectum, very close to the anus. This child has been treated with antibiotics, immune-suppressant medication, and then infliximab, but the abscesses have continued and pro-

gressed. The stricture has gotten worse despite dilation (strictureplas-
ties) by surgeons several times. When the abscesses are present, the
child is in significant pain and is unable to sit up or lie on her back.

Why Surgery Might Be Right for This Child

In this case, the child has very aggressive *perianal* (around the anus)
Crohn disease. Perianal Crohn disease can be very difficult to control
with currently available medical treatments. Furthermore, taking out
the involved parts of intestine is a poor choice because the diseased
areas are so low in the intestines that there is no bowel left to sew the
good intestine to after the removal of the diseased intestine.

The complications of the perianal disease have severely affected
this child's quality of life. As a result, an *intestinal diversion with ostomy*
may be a good option for this child. A diversion surgery involves cutting the intestine above where the severe disease is and bringing that
part of intestine out through an opening in the skin (a stoma). Studies
and experience have shown that moving the contents of the intestines
away from diseased areas allows those areas to heal.

An enterostomal therapist assesses and counsels patients scheduled for diversion surgery. The nurse will tell the child and his family
what to expect from the surgery, will fit the child with the appliance,
and will help prepare everyone for life with the appliance. After the
perianal disease is healed, doctors may decide to perform a *reanastomosis* (hook the intestine back together in normal fashion). However,
the risk of recurrence after reanastomosis remains high, and the right
choice may be to make the stoma permanent.

12
Managing Specific Problems

This chapter describes symptoms of an IBD flare, such as abdominal pain and rectal bleeding, as well as other health problems that a child with IBD may have. We discuss other causes (besides IBD) for each problem as appropriate, and we indicate what action parents might take when these problems occur. Many of the symptoms are also discussed in chapter 4.

Once a child receives a diagnosis of IBD, any new or repeated symptom naturally causes concern that the disease may be "acting up," or flaring. Intestinal symptoms need to be evaluated calmly, to find out whether they are related to IBD or are due to other causes. A child with IBD can get abdominal symptoms (stomachache) for all the same reasons that any child might, reasons such as infections, gas, constipation, and indigestion. If one of your child's friends at school or a family member at home just had a stomach bug, that may be all that is going on.

Abdominal Pain

Abdominal pain is a very common complaint. Once your child reaches an age when she can describe her symptoms, it is always helpful to ask her to describe the pain in her own words. Sometimes the first question to ask is whether your child has felt this type of pain before. Even if she cannot describe it, she can usually answer this question. Children can often distinguish their IBD pain from other types of pain. If they cannot give you a word for the pain, ask about different sensations such as "pressure," "sharp," or "burning." Is the pain there all the time, or does it come and go? Did the pain start suddenly, or come on slowly? If the pain comes and goes, how long does it last each time?

Your child's doctor needs to know where the pain is and how intense it is. He also needs to know if the pain is always in the same place. Crohn disease often involves the area of the intestine that is located in the lower right side, near where most people also know the appendix is located. Pain from the stomach is more likely to be felt in the middle, above the navel (belly button), and pain from the colon is most likely to be felt nearer the middle of the abdomen.

The severity of pain, of course, depends on the person—some people seem to have high tolerance for pain; others are less tolerant. It is helpful to ask the child to compare this pain with past experience. You can also gauge the impact of your child's pain by how much it affects her activity, appetite, or sleep.

Try to determine if the pain is connected with anything. Does it only occur just before a bowel movement? Is it more likely to occur after eating, or with an empty stomach? Are there things that help ease the pain, such as passing gas or stool? In addition, are there things that seem to make the pain worse? Pay particular attention if it seems that coughing or sneezing makes the pain worse. Does the abdomen seem unusually sensitive if you touch or rub it?

Your child may have significant symptoms, such as diarrhea, fever, or vomiting, that the doctor will need to hear about in detail. You should also mention more subtle or seemingly unrelated problems, such as mouth sores, joint pain, fatigue, or weight loss.

Carefully answering these questions will help you and your child's doctor assess how severe and urgent the problem is, and whether immediate medical attention is needed:

- What does the pain feel like (pressure, sharp, burning, etc.)?
- Is the pain constant or does it come and go? For intermittent pain, how long does it last?
- Did the pain start suddenly or slowly?

- Where is the pain located?
- How much does it hurt compared to other abdominal pain in the past?
- Does the pain affect activities of daily living or sleep?
- Does anything make it better or worse?
- Does the pain get worse when the child coughs or sneezes?
- Is the abdomen sensitive to touch?
- Does the child have any other symptoms?

Call your child's doctor if severe, constant pain persists. Call your child's doctor if your child shows signs of unusual sensitivity to touch or motion. Watch to see if milder symptoms go away or continue, especially if they seem different from previous flares of IBD. When in doubt about abdominal pain, it is always best to call your doctor. The nurse or doctor can then help you decide if your child should be seen right away or if any tests should be done.

Rectal Bleeding

Blood in the stool is a common sign that IBD may be flaring. This symptom is never normal, but it is also usually not a reason to panic. Note how much blood is present, how often the child is having a bowel movement, and whether the child has diarrhea. Bloody diarrhea almost always means that the colon is inflamed, and this inflammation can be due to an IBD flare. It is best to contact the doctor early on to rule out infection and decide about further testing and treatment. Rarely, the child may have significant bleeding. *If it seems that there is more blood than stool, seek medical attention immediately.*

If the blood is associated with no change in bowel habits, it may not be due to IBD. Patients in remission may become constipated, and passing hard stool can sometimes cause bleeding from a fissure (small tear or cut in the skin near the anus). People with Crohn disease can also develop inflammation around the anus as part of the disease, and their inflammation can cause bleeding.

Anemia

Persistent loss of blood in the stools (even in tiny or invisible amounts) can lead to low levels of hemoglobin, a condition called anemia. Hemoglobin is the part of the red blood cells that carries oxygen to the rest of the body. Anemia can be caused by direct loss of blood as well as by indirect loss of iron, which is an important part of hemoglobin.

IBD can cause anemia for other reasons in addition to blood loss. Crohn disease of the small intestine may cause iron to be poorly absorbed (taken into the body). The body needs iron to produce new blood cells, and therefore low iron levels can lead to anemia. Other vitamins are also important for the production of blood cells, and poor nutrition or poor absorption of these nutrients (for example, folic acid or vitamin B_{12}) can also lead to anemia.

Mild anemia may not cause any symptoms. As blood counts fall below normal, however, the first symptom you will notice in your child is fatigue (tiredness). More severe anemia can cause dizziness or lightheadedness, shortness of breath, and rapid heart rate. Symptoms will come on more quickly, and be more severe, the faster the blood count falls. During routine visits, as well as during a flare of the disease, the doctor will check your child's blood counts.

Diarrhea

Diarrhea is another common, and often prominent, symptom of IBD, but not every loose stool is cause for concern. Everyone's bowel patterns can change naturally, especially with changes in diet. As with the stomach symptoms discussed earlier in this chapter, take the time to assess exactly what is happening with your child. Until your child has had a few episodes of diarrhea, he may not be able tell how abnormal his stool really is. You may need to insist on seeing it, even if he feels embarrassed by this request.

Make a note of how often the diarrhea occurs, whether it is associated with pain or cramps, and how loose it seems to be. The presence of blood with diarrhea is always an important sign. School-age children typically try not to have bowel movements in school, so if your child begins to have bowel movements at school, that may be a sign of diarrhea. Getting up at night for a bowel movement is a sign of more significant diarrhea. If there is significant diarrhea, bring a stool sample to the doctor's office or clinic. The sample can be checked for hidden blood, then sent to the lab and checked for infection.

Systemic Symptoms

The signs and symptoms of IBD are not always confined to the digestive (gastrointestinal, or GI) tract. Symptoms of IBD may involve the body as a whole, in which case they are called systemic symptoms. Systemic symptoms may include fatigue, loss of appetite with associated weight loss, and fever. Children and adolescents may have delayed growth and delayed puberty.

These problems are largely the result of intestinal inflammation and the related problem of not getting enough calories from food. The immune system releases substances called *cytokines* during inflammation responses. Cytokines cause many systemic signs and symptoms even when the inflammation itself is so mild that there are no obvious GI symptoms.

Fatigue and Loss of Appetite

An important part of maintaining health in a child or adolescent with IBD is identifying and treating specific conditions that can contribute to fatigue, such as anemia (see above) or not eating enough calories. Certain cytokines can reduce appetite, and therefore a person having an inflammation response may not consume enough calories in her diet due to lack of appetite. Inflammation in the stomach (gastritis) can cause discomfort while eating, which again reduces appetite and the amount of food a person eats. Regardless of the cause, if a child is not getting enough calories, the result will be fatigue and weight loss (or poor weight gain), which lead to further harmful effects on a child's health. If a child drinks liquid nutritional supplements during a time of active disease, he will have an easier time maintaining or gaining weight. Controlling the acid in the child's stomach with medications can ease some of the discomfort of eating.

Symptoms such as fatigue and loss of appetite can also be signs of the emotional, psychological (mental), and social effects of this disease, both before and after diagnosis. Fatigue and loss of appetite are common feelings that take a toll on quality of life in anyone with a chronic illness.

Fever

Fevers can be the result of another illness that the child has while also having IBD. This other illness may require specific treatment in addition to the IBD treatment the child is receiving. Fevers associated with IBD are usually low grade and irregular. You can treat them with acetaminophen (for example, Tylenol). Treatment with nonsteroidal anti-inflammatory drugs (NSAIDs) such as ibuprofen (for example, Advil) is controversial and should be avoided when possible for fever. Ibuprofen can worsen IBD and should be taken only on a doctor's advice. These medications can cause additional injury to the digestive tract and may induce an IBD flare.

Delayed Puberty

Disease-related factors can affect growth and puberty (see chapter 4). Some of the most effective medications for treating inflammation—for example, steroids such as prednisone—can slow growth as well. Doctors try very hard to reduce the use of long-term steroids taken by mouth. Treating delayed growth and sexual development involves

- supporting good nutrition,
- treating the inflammation to reduce the release of cytokines, and
- minimizing the use of steroids.

Extraintestinal Manifestations

As discussed in earlier chapters, inflammatory bowel disease affects different portions of the digestive tract. Ulcerative colitis is limited to the large intestine, and Crohn disease can affect any area between the mouth and the anus. However, it is not unusual for other parts of the body to be affected by IBD as well. When the disease involves areas beyond the digestive tract, the problems created by the IBD are called *extraintestinal manifestations* of inflammatory bowel disease. Some of these extraintestinal manifestations occur only when digestive tract inflammation is active, while others occur when there are no digestive tract symptoms. The following sections discuss some of the extra-intestinal manifestations of IBD.

Joints and Bones

Many children have joint pain (*arthralgia*) and arm and leg (extremity) pain, whether or not the child has IBD. "Growing pains" are a common part of normal childhood, as are other causes of joint and bone pain, such as sports injuries. Nonetheless, extremity and joint pain can be specifically related to IBD or to the medications used to treat IBD. Joint pain can occur when the doctor decreases prednisone doses, or when a child starts taking immunosuppressant medications, such as aza-thioprine or 6-mercaptopurine. Joint pain associated with medication changes usually goes away over time and does not require treatment.

Joint inflammation (*arthritis*) occurs in up to 20 percent of adults with IBD, but it seems to affect children and teens less commonly. In contrast to joint pain, arthritis causes not only pain but also joint swelling and redness, and the joint might feel warm to the touch. Despite these symptoms, the types of arthritis associated with IBD rarely damage the affected joints. Nevertheless, you should *notify your child's IBD specialist immediately if a joint becomes red and swollen*, because it is important to rule out an infection in the joint. Depending on the type and severity of the arthritis, the doctor may want your child to be seen by a pediatric rheumatologist, an expert in children with arthritis.

Some types of IBD-related arthritis worsen only when the digestive tract symptoms worsen. In those cases, treating the digestive tract symptoms also effectively treats the arthritis. Pain medications with or without physical therapy may be prescribed while the digestive tract symptoms are treated. In cases where the arthritis occurs without digestive tract symptoms, treatment may involve physical therapy, pain medication, and medicines such as steroids, methotrexate, or infliximab to suppress the inflammation.

Ibuprofen and similar medicines to treat pain can worsen IBD, but some doctors will suggest trying these medications and continuing them if digestive tract symptoms do not worsen. You should discuss the risks and benefits of using ibuprofen and related pain-relief medications with your child's physician.

Rarely, the joints of the back can be affected by IBD in conditions called *sacroiliitis* and *ankylosing spondylitis*. Symptoms of these disorders include morning back stiffness, gradual low back pain that is worse with rest, and pain spreading to the buttocks. These problems can occur even when there are no digestive tract symptoms. Should these symptoms develop, your child's IBD specialist may order x-rays and blood tests. Treatment of ankylosing spondylitis and sacroiliitis may include pain medications and immunosuppressant medications such as methotrexate and infliximab. Your child's doctor will probably want your child to be examined by a pediatric rheumatologist.

Decreased bone density, called *osteopenia,* and a more severe condition, *osteoporosis,* is common in adults with IBD and can occur in children and adolescents with IBD as well. Considerably decreased bone density can increase the risk of broken bones (fractures). It is likely that many different factors affect bone density in IBD. Although more research is needed, factors thought to decrease bone density include

- steroid use
- insufficient calcium and vitamin D in the diet
- problems with absorption of calcium and vitamin D (the child gets enough calcium and vitamin D in the diet, but the body can't take it in and use it because the intestinal lining is damaged)

- inactivity
- alcohol use
- smoking
- digestive tract inflammation

The best way to prevent osteoporosis in children with IBD is still unknown. Getting enough calcium and vitamin D in the diet, avoiding alcohol and tobacco, and exercising regularly are all recommended. If your child has severe or persistent bone or back pain, you should notify the IBD specialist. An x-ray or other tests may be needed. Some doctors recommend tests to screen for osteoporosis as part of routine care, while others do so only in specific situations.

Mouth and Skin

Mouth sores or mouth ulcers are common in children and adolescents with IBD, and many healthy children have them, too. In children with IBD, they tend to worsen during flares of digestive tract symptoms and improve when the digestive tract symptoms are treated. They may also go away without any particular treatment. Although the condition is generally more of an annoyance than a serious complication, mouth pain from the ulcers may cause children to eat poorly. Topical numbing mouthwashes can help decrease the discomfort associated with mouth sores and may make eating easier. Your child's doctor may recommend other medications or mouthwashes, if the topical numbing washes are not enough.

Rashes such as eczema, dry skin, and acne are common in children with and without IBD. Steroids may make acne worse in adolescents. In addition to these normal childhood rashes, children with IBD are at risk for other skin problems as well, such as erythema nodosum and pyoderma gangrenosum. Both are relatively uncommon, particularly in children.

Erythema nodosum typically appears as red, painful bumps on the front of the lower legs. It tends to occur when digestive tract symptoms flare, and it goes away either on its own, or as the digestive tract symptoms are treated.

Pyoderma gangrenosum begins as pustules (pus-filled bumps), often on the feet or lower legs. The pustules then develop into skin ulcerations. Ulcerations are usually painful, and they can be brought on or worsened by injury to the skin. They can occur without any digestive tract symptoms. While they may go away on their own over a period of several months, they are often treated with immunosuppressant medications such as steroids, cyclosporine (or related medications), or infliximab.

As explained elsewhere in this book, Crohn disease often results in fissures, ulcers, and tags (thickened flaps of skin), mostly on the skin around the anus. Occasionally, similar problems occur on the skin of other areas of the body. This condition is referred to as *metastatic cutaneous* Crohn disease. Metastatic cutaneous Crohn disease can occur even when digestive tract symptoms are absent. Treatment of this condition often involves taking one or more immunosuppressant medications.

Eyes

We mentioned eye problems in chapter 4. Eye problems are often treated with eye drops, but oral steroids or immunosuppressant medications may occasionally be needed. Steroids can cause other eye problems, such as glaucoma or cataracts, when used for long periods.

Liver Disease

This discussion provides information on the treatment of the liver conditions mentioned in chapter 4. A doctor may suspect liver disease when a child's liver function tests are abnormal. Liver function tests are blood tests that measure levels of certain liver enzymes such as GGT, ALT, and AST. Another liver function test measures the level of bilirubin, a product of the breakdown of red blood cells (red blood cells are broken down in the liver).

To treat primary sclerosing cholangitis (PSC, inflammation of the bile ducts), doctors may prescribe ursodeoxycholate (ursodiol). Other anti-inflammatory and immunosuppressive treatments are sometimes used, but none has been conclusively proven to work. Some patients with severe PSC may need a liver transplant.

Gallstones often do not cause symptoms, and if any are found during an ultrasound, they do not need to be treated. Rarely, they may "get stuck" and cause symptoms in a bile duct, and then they need to be removed through an ERCP scope (see chapter 9). If inflammation of the gallbladder develops (if the child has a "gallbladder attack"), the gallbladder (often with gallstones inside) will need to be surgically removed. This surgery can be done safely through a laparoscopy in almost all patients, even after surgery for CD. A laparoscopy is surgery through the belly button; it involves smaller incisions (cuts) and quicker recovery than laparotomy. Because the gallbladder stores, concentrates, and releases bile, removing bile after surgery may require more frequent, smaller meals that are low in fat to avoid diarrhea.

Fatty liver disease (*nonalcoholic steatohepatitis,* or NASH, or nonalcoholic fatty liver disease, or NAFLD) can occur with extended use of steroids, severe or sudden weight gain or weight loss, or too much *total parenteral nutrition,* or TPN (intravenous nutrition). The liver may become enlarged, with abnormal collections of fat inside the liver cells. NASH usually clears if a person

- follows a healthy diet
- takes ursodiol and vitamin E
- decreases steroid use
- reaches and maintains a normal weight

If NASH is severe or longstanding, however, cirrhosis and its complications can occur, though this is rare. Cirrhosis is scarring of the liver, which causes permanent liver damage.

Medications used to treat IBD, including azathioprine and 6-MP, can cause *drug-related hepatitis* (inflammation of the liver) in some children, due to individual differences in how the body processes these drugs. If your child develops hepatitis while taking any of these medicines, the doctor may decrease the dose or stop that particular medicine altogether. People taking these medications should have their medication levels and liver functions regularly monitored by their physician. This is done through blood tests.

A medicine related to azathioprine and 6-MP, called 6-thioguanine (6-TG), has been linked with a rare but possibly permanent liver disease called vaso-occlusive disease (VOD). The use of this medicine should probably be avoided in children with IBD.

Kidney Problems

IBD is associated with a greater than average risk of developing certain kidney diseases. People with Crohn disease, especially those whose bodies malabsorb fat, may develop kidney stones. (Fat malabsorption occurs when the body cannot take in the fat that a person eats.) These stones may cause no symptoms, but sometimes they cause severe pain, blood in the urine, and decreased urination due to obstruction. Kidney stones may also damage the kidneys. Maintaining good control of Crohn disease, eating a healthy low-fat diet, and drinking lots of water (to avoid dehydration) helps prevent kidney stones. If they develop, there are different approaches to treating them. Stones sometimes pass out of the body on their own (in the urine), but if they do not, then medications can be taken or the stones can be removed by inserting an endoscope through an incision (in keyhole surgery) or using lithotripsy. Lithotripsy is a noninvasive procedure done while the patient is sedated or under anesthesia. A focused, high-intensity acoustic pulse is applied through the skin in an attempt to break up the stones, to make them small enough to pass out of the body through the ureters.

Cyclosporine and tacrolimus are medications that a doctor might prescribe to treat severe ulcerative colitis and, though rarely, severe Crohn disease. These medicines directly damage the kidneys, especially at higher doses or if they are used for a long time. Individuals taking these medications must take them *exactly* as they have been prescribed and must have regular blood tests to check the level of the medication in the blood and to check kidney function. Careful monitoring is needed to avoid permanent kidney damage, high blood pressure, and kidney failure. A person with kidney failure requires dialysis or a kidney transplant.

Some people with IBD have an increased risk of developing a form of kidney inflammation called *tubular interstitial nephritis* that can cause the kidneys to stop working. Medications containing 5-aminosalicylates (5-ASA), such as mesalamine, olsalazine, balsalazide and sulfasalazine, can increase the risk of developing this problem. Although most doctors do not routinely check blood levels of these medications, people taking these medications should have regular urinalysis and blood tests to check creatinine levels (a kidney function test). If abnormalities are found, patients should stop taking the medicines in order to prevent permanent kidney damage.

Rarely, during a difficult pelvic surgery for UC, such as a pouch procedure, the ureters (the tubes connecting the kidney to the bladder) are damaged. If this happens, the ureters will require surgical repair. During this surgery there may also be damage to the nerves of the bladder or the urogenital system. This nerve damage can lead to urinary incontinence or impotence (in males). This surgical complication is rare, but it is a recognized risk and is not always correctable if it occurs.

Bladder Problems

Crohn disease can affect the bladder. When patients experience the symptoms of urinary tract infection—pain or a burning sensation during urination—the cause of these symptoms may be irritation from an adjacent inflamed part of the bowel or a fistula connecting the intestine to the bladder. When a patient has irritation, a urine test may reveal an increase in white blood cells (the cells that are involved in the inflammatory process and in fighting infections). In irritation, no bacteria are found in a urine test. When a patient has a fistula, a urine test may reveal air, blood, and even small remains of stool as well as bacteria.

In people with Crohn disease, a fistula (abnormal opening) sometimes develops between the digestive tract and the bladder, which can lead to infection. Radiographic studies such as abdominal CT scan or magnetic resonance imaging (MRI) may identify the fistula. Surgery may be necessary to treat this complication of the disease.

In many patients with a fistula to the bladder, urinary tract infections tend to come back, but serious complications, such as kidney infections, are very rare. A fistula can be identified by a barium x-ray, by a CT scan, or by a direct examination of the bladder by a physician looking through a cystoscope (a device similar to the endoscope but with a very slim tube).

Antibiotics and anti-inflammatory medicines (such as steroids or azathioprine) may be effective in treating bladder problems. When a fistula is present, or when symptoms do not go away with medical therapy, surgical removal of the inflamed part of the bowel, and the fistula, will solve the problem. Special diets are not very helpful in the treatment of these problems.

Strictures

Strictures, or narrowing of the bowel due to inflammation and scarring, are very common in CD. Strictures may cause no symptoms and be discovered only during a barium test (see chapter 8). Strictures can cause symptoms, however, including cramping pain, bloating, nausea, vomiting, and less frequent and less satisfactory bowel movements. These symptoms result when the flow of intestinal contents is blocked. If these symptoms occur, let the doctor know immediately. Rarely, infection and reduced blood flow to the bowel can result from strictures, and these problems require medication or surgery.

For an acute obstruction, usually a short period of bowel "rest" (no food or drink by mouth), intravenous fluids, and steroids relieve stricture-related obstruction without the need for surgery to remove the affected area, although surgery may sometimes be necessary. If the narrowed area is within the reach of an endoscope, the doctor may place a stent or inject steroids directly into the stricture to try to prevent a return of the problem. If the stricture is long, surgery to widen the opening through the intestine (called strictureplasty) can be done, often laparoscopically (through the belly button). Doctors recommend this surgery to relieve the symptoms of chronic or recurrent obstruction, while avoiding the possible loss of too much bowel. (Losing too much bowel can lead to a problem known as *short bowel syndrome.*)

If your child has strictures, the following tips can help reduce her risk of obstruction:

- Avoid high-roughage foods like nuts and popcorn.
- Chew food completely.
- Drink plenty of fluids with meals.
- Eat smaller meals more frequently.
- Avoid capsule endoscopy (pill camera, see chapter 8), because the camera capsule can get stuck.

Abscess

An abscess, or local infection, is rare in people with UC but is more common in people with CD. Symptoms vary by the site of the abscess. They include fever, chills, lethargy, and pain. Other symptoms include tenderness, redness, and warmth in the area or the skin above it, as well as drainage (oozing). If these symptoms occur, tell your doctor immediately because sepsis, a severe bodywide infection in the bloodstream, may occur. A CT scan or MRI scan (see chapter 8) may help diagnose an abscess if it is in the abdomen or pelvis, and blood tests often show an elevated white blood cell count. (An elevated white blood cell count indicates an infection.)

People who have recently had surgery or other procedures, or people who have a fistula, are at higher risk of getting an abscess. Another risk factor is taking medications that suppress the immune system, especially taking these medications at high doses or for long periods. People with suppressed immune systems may have more subtle signs of an abscess at first, but they may get sicker from it.

If your child has an abscess, the doctor may put him on antibiotics by mouth or by IV (through the vein). In some cases, a surgeon may have to drain the abscess. A radiologist with a needle guided by ultrasound or CT scan can also drain an abscess. When an abscess affects the skin, wound care experts may provide additional advice. Keeping the area clean, dry, and protected often helps with healing.

Fistula

Fistula, an abnormal opening or connection between the digestive tract and other organs, typically occurs in CD. Only very rarely do fistulas develop in people with UC, most often after pouch surgery. If a fistula happens after pouch surgery, pouch correction and removal (resulting in the need for permanent ileostomy; see chapter 11) are frequently required.

A fistula can also result from or lead to infection, including the development of an abscess. Symptoms of fistula vary greatly, as do the treatment options and the success of treatment. Symptoms and treatments of fistulas depend on their location, number, and size, as well as on how long the fistula was present before treatment and whether it is internal (inside the body) or external (opens onto the skin).

In CD, fistulas from the intestine to the skin and tissues around the anus are common and are easier to treat than other fistulas. Symptoms include pain, irritation, and swelling. Drainage of stool, blood, and pus can occur, making sitting and walking uncomfortable.

Pain control is an important part of treating fistulas. There are many new and improved treatments available. Antibiotics (ciprofloxacin and metronidazole) are effective in decreasing symptoms and healing fistula, but when these treatments stop, recurrence is common. Once any infection is cleared, antibiotic therapy may be followed by infliximab, or by cyclosporine or tacrolimus. The surgeon may place a seton (a piece of fabric, thread, or a small plastic wick) in the fistulous tract to promote healing, particularly in patients with an abscess. Fibrin "glue" can also help close the opening.

It is not always possible to achieve lasting healing of the fistula, even with infliximab, the most effective therapy. Incomplete closure may be acceptable if a person is otherwise doing well. Once closed, continuous treatment with infliximab, 6-MP, or azathioprine will likely be required to prevent recurrence.

Diagnosis of other types of fistulas can be difficult and requires a combination of tests including barium x-rays, CT scan, MRI, ultrasound, and endoscopy or colonoscopy. These tests may require anesthesia to avoid discomfort. Very rarely, a fistula develops that connects the rectum and the vagina, or other organs of the reproductive tract, including the fallopian tubes and ovary. These types of fistulas are particularly difficult to treat and potentially very harmful socially. They can also cause severe problems when a woman tries to become pregnant. A stoma (see chapter 11) or many surgeries, combined with medications, are often necessary to treat fistulas involving the reproductive organs.

Internal fistulas from one diseased bowel area to another may not cause any symptoms and may not require treatment. Surgery to remove the connected segments may be needed, however, if symptoms occur or if the fistula connects to the bladder or the urinary tract, causing repeated infections.

Perforation

A perforation of the intestines occurs when the wall of the intestines develops a hole, allowing the contents of the intestines (especially bacteria) to spill into nearby spaces and organs. A perforation may result in the formation of an abscess (see above) or in a more general infection of the abdominal cavity (called *peritonitis*). A perforation causing a localized abscess is called a *walled-off perforation*. This happens when a nearby structure (such as the intestine itself, the bladder, or the uterus) seals off the perforation. A perforation resulting in peritonitis is called a *free perforation*.

Free perforations are uncommon in IBD. In Crohn disease, perforations usually occur in the small bowel, are generally walled off, and may be the first symptom of the disease. In ulcerative colitis, free perforations can occur in the large bowel (colon) and are likely to cause peritonitis.

The main risk factors leading to perforations are severe inflammation and enlarged segments of bowel that are ahead of a stricture.

Your child's doctor will suspect a perforation if your child suddenly develops abdominal tenderness, pain, and fever. A new mass (lump), detected during a physical exam, can also be a sign of perforation.

When the doctor suspects a perforation, he will order tests such as abdominal x-ray, ultrasound, CT scan, or MRI of the abdomen to examine the intestine and the abdominal area. If the doctor finds a perforation, treatment will usually begin with antibiotics to control any possible infection. When there is a free perforation, immediate surgery may be required to seal it off. In these cases, it is likely that no food by mouth will be allowed until the child recovers from the surgery, and feeding will be done through a vein.

When the child has a walled-off perforation, surgery may be required to either drain the abscess or remove the diseased portion of intestine. The timing of the surgery will depend on the response to treatment. If the child is having severe pain with regular diet, switching to a liquid formula may help.

IBD experts believe that perforation is a feature of a subgroup of Crohn disease. Patients with this type of Crohn disease are at higher risk of repeated fistulas or perforation. At present, there is no known way to prevent this complication.

Cancer

One of the long-term complications of IBD is colon cancer, which is tied to the chronic inflammation of the colon. The risk of developing colon cancer depends on how long the person has had IBD and how severe the inflammation of the colon is. The risk increases beyond the risk of the general population once a person has had the disease for more than eight years. Experts say that once a person has had ulcerative colitis for ten years, the risk of cancer goes up by about 0.5 percent each year. There are not as much data for Crohn disease, but the risk may be comparable to UC if the extent and duration of colon inflammation is similar. The cancer risk does not go away even if the disease remains inactive (in remission), but there is some evidence that keeping the disease in remission can help decrease the risk.

Taking this risk into account, once the disease has been present for eight to ten years, regular screening for colon cancer must begin. Most children with IBD are diagnosed in their teens, so this concern does not often come up until the college years or early adulthood. Monitoring includes annual checkups with a gastroenterologist and regular colonoscopies with biopsies to look for the early signs of cancer.

Researchers are constantly looking for new, less-invasive ways to detect cancer early. It is likely that in the not-too-distant future, we will monitor for cancer by testing blood or stool, instead of with a colonoscopy. CT scans and MRI imaging are already nearly as effective at detecting polyps and colon cancer as a colonoscopy. As new testing becomes available, the screening recommendations will change.

13

The Role of Nutrition

Just as a builder must have tools to make a house, children's bodies must have food to help them grow and to give them energy to play and do schoolwork. When children are sick, food becomes even more important, because good nutrition is necessary to help them get better.

Doctors and dieticians often use the word *nutrition* when they talk about the benefits of food. Nutrition includes proteins, carbohydrates, fats, and other important materials such as vitamins and minerals. When your child has inflammatory bowel disease, she needs good nutrition to get better. Your child's doctor will recommend many helpful and healthy foods for your child. If your child cannot eat all of the recommended foods, the doctor will suggest some nutritional supplements.

The first symptoms of IBD in children and adolescents often include weight loss or failure to gain weight at a normal rate. Many people who have IBD find it difficult to eat enough good food. They may feel hungry, but when it is time to eat, they can finish only a small amount. Food may not taste good, or they may just find it difficult to eat. Some people get stomachaches or diarrhea after eating, so they stop eating in order to avoid these symptoms.

An inflamed, swollen portion of the intestine acts like a funnel through which food and gas must pass. As they pass, the thickened (and sometimes ulcerated) bowel stretches, causing pain or other unpleasant symptoms. By eating less, children decrease the food-related symptoms. For those with Crohn disease, a severe narrowing of the gut can cause even worse symptoms.

If a child does not eat well for a long time, weight loss, slow growth, and delayed sexual development can result. In addition, intestinal inflammation symptoms can become worse when a person does not eat, because the body lacks the building blocks necessary to heal the intestine.

Nutrition is important to your child's whole body, including the digestive tract—the mouth, stomach, and small and large intestines. Therefore, most doctors try to supply the gastrointestinal (GI) tract with nutrients. In the past, doctors thought that not putting any food in the GI tract would help it heal by giving it a rest, and they would prescribe that the child have nothing to eat (but plenty of fluids) for

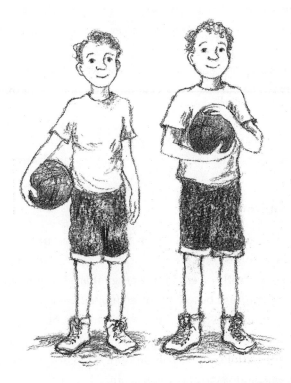

Treatment and control of inflammatory bowel disease often results in improvement in weight, height, and muscle mass. This picture shows what a difference treatment can make. On the left is the child before treatment, and on the right the same child is shown after treatment.

several weeks. They found, however, that the digestive tract needs food just as much as the rest of the body. Doctors no longer prescribe "bowel rest" except in rare situations.

Because of the eating and nutrition problems of people with IBD, the doctor may pay special attention to your child's bones. Normally, bones become stronger as a child grows and continue to get stronger until a person reaches his mid-twenties. Several factors, however, can cause people with IBD to have weaker bones than normal:

- Children with IBD may not get enough minerals, such as calcium and phosphorus, and vitamins, such as vitamin D. This occurs for two reasons: they are not consuming adequate amounts, and they may have some degree of malabsorption. These minerals and vitamins are necessary for strong, healthy bones.
- Some medications, such as steroids, can weaken bones. Your child may need to take extra vitamins and minerals for their bones.

The doctor may request a special test for your child, to check bone strength. The test is called DEXA (dual-energy x-ray absorptiometry).

Caloric Requirements

According to some reports, children with IBD symptoms eat only about half the calories they require for their age. Children and teens with IBD need 20 to 40 percent more energy than children who do not have IBD. This figure is based on the estimated energy requirements (EER) for healthy children. The EER is the amount of energy that the Food and Nutrition Board considers sufficient to meet the known needs of most healthy people. This amount will vary depending on a child's size, age, and stage of development.

As a rough estimate, children with IBD need about 2,000 to 2,200 calories every day for girls, and 2,300 to 2,600 calories every day for boys. Your doctor will tell you what your child's calorie needs are, or your doctor may ask a dietician to help you figure out how many calories your child needs. The dietician can show you what foods will help give your child the calories she needs.

Protein and calories work together. Your child needs the right combination of both. For growing children and teens with inflammatory bowel disease, the protein requirements range from 2.4 to 3.0 grams per kilogram (kg) of body weight, per day (1 kg = 2.2 lbs). For example, a child who weighs 90 pounds needs 98 to 123 grams of protein daily.

Medications that undo the inflammation increase the width of the gut, allowing food to pass more easily. When treatment starts, some children find it easier to eat several small meals and snacks in a day, rather than three regular meals. Making sure that a child gets enough calories and protein to continue growing is more important than the number of meals a child eats. The recommended goals for weight gain will depend on the child's age, sex, and degree of undernutrition.

Specific Nutrients

Iron

Apart from overall inadequate caloric intake, the most common nutritional problem for children and teenagers with IBD is iron deficiency. Iron deficiency can lead to anemia (low red blood cell count). This deficiency occurs for a number of reasons in people with IBD, including not getting enough iron from food, decreased iron absorption in the gut, and increased iron losses from the intestine due to visible bleeding or hidden (*occult*) bleeding. Doctors usually diagnose iron deficiency anemia in a routine blood test and treat the anemia with iron supplements.

Calcium

Calcium is an essential part of bones. Along with phosphorus, it gives bone its strength. Calcium plays very important roles in passing nerve signals along and in muscle contraction.

All people with IBD, and especially growing children, must consume their daily requirement of calcium. This will help ensure the normal development of their bones and prevent osteoporosis in the future. Calcium requirements change with age and are highest in children entering puberty, a time when they are growing fast. There are several guidelines for calcium requirements in children. In general, for children between ages 1 and 9, 500 to 800 mg of calcium per day is recommended, whereas children aged 9 to 18 years should get 1,200 to 1,300 mg each day.

Calcium occurs naturally in a variety of foods, and most people with IBD can absorb calcium normally from the intestine. The most important dietary source of calcium is dairy products. One cup of milk or yogurt contains 300 mg of calcium, and 1 ounce of natural or processed cheese has 200 mg of calcium. Other foods that contain calcium, although less of it, are

- canned fish with bones (250 mg in 3 oz)
- corn tortillas
- calcium-set tofu
- Chinese cabbage
- kale
- broccoli

Some people reduce their intake of dairy and calcium because of symptoms of lactose intolerance (inability to digest foods containing lactose). To avoid this problem, they can choose lactose-free products and dairy products that have low lactose content and still have a good level of calcium. These include aged cheeses, cottage cheese, kefir cultured milk drink, processed and natural cheeses, and yogurt with live cultures. Many juices are now fortified with calcium and offer an alternative to milk as a source of calcium (they contain 320 mg of calcium in each cup). Soda and other soft drinks do not contain calcium. Individuals who drink soda instead of milk may not get enough calcium in their diet.

Some medications used to treat IBD, especially corticosteroids, can affect the absorption of calcium, and when used long term, they can

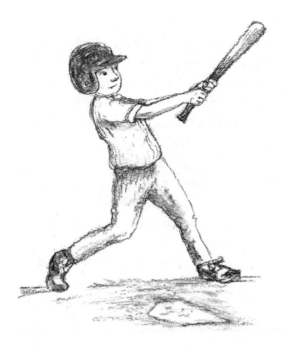

affect bone strength. Although corticosteroids are excellent medications to bring about remission in IBD, they do not work well to maintain remission. Therefore, after your child feels better, the doctor will use medications that offer the possibility of long-term remission without the unwelcome side effects of corticosteroids. This approach should help minimize the effect of corticosteroids on bone health as well. If your child cannot stop taking corticosteroids, taking them every other day will minimize their side effects while maintaining their benefits.

Several national campaigns are designed to encourage adequate calcium intake in growing children and teens. Reliable information on this subject can be obtained from the report on the following Web site: www.surgeongeneral.gov/topics/bonehealth.

Lactose

Lactose is the sugar found in the milk of mammals. It is found in human and cow's milk and in any dairy products derived from milk.

Lactose intolerance is a condition where eating or drinking something that contains lactose causes abdominal pain, diarrhea, or gas. These symptoms occur when someone does not have enough *lactase*, the intestinal enzyme that digests (breaks down) lactose. An intestinal enzyme is a special type of protein located on the lining of the intestines.

Many people think they should avoid lactose if they have IBD. Studies have shown, however, that lactose intolerance is no more prevalent among people with IBD than among people without IBD. Therefore, your child should not restrict dairy products unless he has proven lactose intolerance. Even then, studies show that most people with real lactose intolerance can drink about 8 ounces of milk (1 cup) without having symptoms.

If your child has lactose intolerance and drinks lactose, it will not harm his body. He may experience loose stools or some gas and abdominal discomfort, but these symptoms will stop in an hour or two. Tablets that contain lactase (the enzyme that breaks down milk sugar) can be taken to help minimize or eliminate the symptoms that might otherwise occur. Your child can take the tablets (pills) before eating or drinking foods that contain lactose. Your child can also drink milk that is treated with the enzyme lactase to remove lactose (for example, Lactaid milk).

If you think your child has symptoms with lactose ingestion, ask his doctor about available tests to diagnose lactose intolerance. Sometimes it is difficult to eliminate all dairy products from a diet without the help of a dietician. There is no reason to deny your child desirable dairy food if he or she is not lactose intolerant.

Fiber

Fiber is made of plant materials that humans cannot digest. It helps normal bowel movements and helps prevent diseases such as cancer, heart disease, obesity, and diabetes. Unfortunately, most Americans do not eat enough fiber. Unless your child's doctor thinks your child should not have fiber, there is no reason to limit fiber-containing foods just because your child has IBD. The National Academy of Sciences recommends that children between the ages of 9 and 18 have 29 to 38 grams of fiber every day.

Vitamin D

Vitamin D helps the body absorb calcium in the intestine. The body produces vitamin D naturally when the skin is exposed to sunlight. The daily requirement of vitamin D is 400 IU (international units) each day or 800 IU each day when exposure to sunlight is limited. Few foods are a natural source of vitamin D; some foods are fortified (have added vitamin D).

Foods that naturally contain vitamin D include fish liver oils, flesh of fatty fish (such as salmon and herring), and eggs (from hens that have been fed vitamin D). In the United States, milk is fortified with vitamin D (400 IU/quart), and cereals are also fortified.

Vitamin D production in the skin is the body's major natural source of this important nutrient. Natural sunlight stimulates the production of vitamin D in the skin. Children who do not feel well and stay indoors a lot are at risk for vitamin D deficiency. In addition, children living in northern areas have lower vitamin D levels in the fall and winter, due to lack of exposure to sunlight.

Skin protected by sunblock lotions or creams will produce only a little vitamin D. Exposure to sunlight shining through glass windows is not enough to stimulate vitamin D production in the skin. Only sensible exposure of unprotected skin to natural sunlight can ensure an adequate supply of this vitamin. In general, however, using sunblock is recommended to protect against skin cancer.

Folic Acid

Folic acid is a form of vitamin B. Sources of folic acid include

- enriched cereal grains
- dark leafy vegetables
- enriched and whole-grain breads and bread products
- fortified ready-to-eat cereals

People who do not have enough folic acid (folic acid deficiency) may develop anemia (low number of red blood cells). People with IBD who take sulfasalazine (a medication that treats colon inflammation) can develop folic acid deficiency. Daily folic acid supplements, given in tablet (pill) form, can correct this deficiency. These tablets are available over the counter. Folic acid should also be given to anyone receiving methotrexate treatment.

Folic acid may play a role in reducing long-term colon cancer risk in people with IBD (particularly ulcerative colitis), although more studies are needed on this subject. Another possible benefit of folic acid supplements may be a decrease in homocysteine levels. Homocysteine is a chemical that has been linked to cardiovascular (heart) disease and to the risk of thrombosis (blood clots).

Vitamin B12

Vitamin B_{12} is found in fortified cereals, meat, fish, and poultry; it is specifically absorbed in the lower ileum (the ileum is the last part of the small intestine). Patients with IBD who have inflamed lower ileum (*ileitis*), or who have had surgery to remove this part of their intestines, are at risk for vitamin B_{12} deficiency. Prolonged vitamin B_{12} deficiency leads to anemia and nerve damage. This deficiency can take months or years to develop because the body stores a large amount of vitamin B_{12} in the liver. It takes time to exhaust this supply. The doctor can measure the amount of vitamin B_{12} in your child's body with a blood test. This will determine if your child needs vitamin B_{12} supplements. A vitamin B_{12} gel given into the nose, or monthly injections of vitamin B_{12}, can correct a deficiency if it develops.

Zinc

Zinc is another important element for the body. Zinc is necessary to help your child grow normally, and for her body to heal. It may even protect against infections. Zinc is lost in diarrhea; the more diarrhea your child has, the more zinc she will lose. Your child's doctor may check blood for zinc levels and, depending on the result, recommend that she take a zinc supplement.

Other Vitamins and Minerals

Many specialists recommend that children with IBD take multivitamin and mineral supplements daily because of reports of certain vitamin and mineral deficiencies in children with this disease. For example, one out of eight children with IBD has a deficiency in vitamin A and vitamin E. Oral vitamin supplements can correct or prevent these deficiencies in most people.

Some studies suggest that children with IBD may benefit from taking antioxidants such as vitamin E, although more studies are needed to confirm whether there is a real benefit to this supplement.

Vitamin K, an important factor in normal blood clotting, is also active in bone. Mild vitamin K deficiency may play a role in bone loss in IBD.

Children with IBD may also have mineral deficiencies, especially during disease exacerbations (worsening). For example, people with chronic diarrhea may lose potassium and magnesium in their stool. Someone with a shortened gut after surgical removal of the intestines is at risk for electrolyte imbalances. Electrolytes are minerals dissolved in body fluids. The body needs electrolytes. Electrolytes can often be replaced by consuming specialized fluids that contain sodium and potassium, such as Gatorade or Pedialyte.

Special Nutritional Formula

We know that nutritional status, particularly not getting enough nutrition, complicates the course of inflammatory bowel disease and changes the effectiveness of treatments. If your child has trouble getting enough food by mouth and is unable to keep up normal body functions (including a normal growth and immune response), he needs to be fed through other means. Nutritional support can be beneficial for a child with either ulcerative colitis or Crohn disease, especially if the child is not growing enough, or is undernourished.

In ulcerative colitis, *enteral nutrition* is usually a supplement to the child's regular diet. Enteral nutrition helps the child either catch up on lost weight or keep himself well nourished through a period of serious illness. Nutritional support can also be one form of treatment for children with Crohn disease.

Enteral Nutrition Support

Enteral nutrition can be taken by mouth, but repeatedly drinking the same liquid foods (formulas) may become tedious or difficult for a child. In these situations, tube feedings are an alternative way to provide the formulas that have all the nutrition your child needs to get better. Best of all, tube feedings can be done overnight. Many people find it reassuring to receive all the nutrition they need while they sleep. They are then free during the day to join their friends and family at the table without worrying about eating more than they feel they can. The tube delivers the formula directly into the intestinal tract (including the stomach or the first part of the small intestine, just past the stomach; figure 13.1). It is an important treatment option that is available to all people with inflammatory bowel disease.

A tube that starts in the nose and goes into the stomach (known as a *nasogastric tube,* or *NG tube*) can deliver enteral nutrition support, and so can a tube that starts in the nose and goes into the small intestine (called a *nasojejunal tube,* or *NJ tube*). A tube that is surgically placed directly into the stomach (*gastrostomy tube,* or *G tube*) or into the small intestine (*jejunostomy tube,* or *J tube*) can also deliver this type of nutrition (table 13.1). Each route of entry into the gastrointestinal system has its advantages and disadvantages.

A tube placed through the nose is initially more uncomfortable. Children resist the insertion of the tube, sometimes making it more difficult to put it into the stomach. Once in place, the tube tends to cause some discomfort and irritation in the back of the nose and throat. Nonetheless, most children who decide to use this treatment

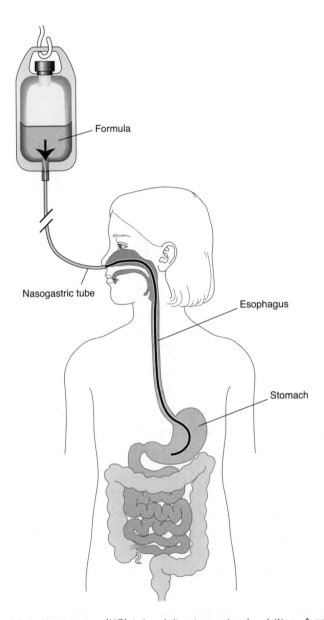

Figure 13.1. Nasogastric (NG) tube delivering enteral nutrition. A patient receiving enteral nutrition learns to pass a small flexible tube past their nasal cavity and esophagus and into the stomach. The tube can then be used to deliver supplemental formula. The formula is sometimes delivered at night by a small pump while the patient is asleep.

Table 13.1. Types of tubes for enteral nutrition

Tube type	Abbreviation	Location
Nasogastric	NG	Tube is in the nose and goes into the stomach
Nasojejunal	NJ	Tube is in the nose and goes to second part of the small intestine (jejunum)
Gastrostomy	G tube	Tube is in the wall of the abdomen and leads into the stomach
Jejunostomy	J tube	Tube is in the wall of the abdomen and leads into the jejunum

adapt, and within a few minutes or hours, they accept the tube and move on to other activities. Often children will place NG tubes into their stomach at night prior to going to bed, thus using the tube and obtaining the extra nutrition while asleep, and then removing the tube in the morning when they wake up. This way, they can go to school and participate in other activities without the tube in place.

An NJ tube placed through the nose into the middle of the small intestine (jejunum) is more difficult to manage. Making sure the tube is in the proper position often involves an x-ray. The x-ray helps to make sure the tube is in the intestine and not in the stomach. Therefore, the NJ tube cannot be removed daily as an NG tube can. Despite good positioning within the intestine, NJ tubes may come back into the stomach. Children might even vomit out the tube, and then the tube must be replaced.

Doctors can insert tubes surgically through the skin and muscles of the abdominal wall, directly into the stomach or small intestine. That way, the tube does not have to pass down from the nose. Stomach tubes are usually placed by endoscopy in a 20-minute procedure called *percutaneous endoscopic gastrostomy* (PEG). The PEG procedure is relatively safe. Most of the time, a small tube that is almost flat to the skin of the abdomen can be used, although sometimes a longer tube is needed. The tubes are fairly easy to change when needed, which may be every two to six months (or longer). Tubes are changed when they break, or when they become too tight and a larger size is needed.

Tubes that pass through the nose are kept in place with tape or other types of adhesives. If they slip out, the tube should be repositioned or completely replaced. Gastrostomy and jejunostomy tubes remain in place by a balloon or plastic dome within the stomach or intestine. The balloon can inadvertently deflate, and the tube may come out. Should this happen, the tube should be replaced immediately so that the hole into the stomach or into the jejunum does not close. If the tube is difficult to replace or cannot be replaced, then your physician should be notified, and your child should be seen in the emergency room.

Once a tube is in place and provides access to the intestinal tract, it can be used for nourishment. Sometimes the tube is used only for giving medication or fluid (such as water). In most cases of inflammatory bowel disease, however, the tube is used for formula feeding. The formula is given through the tube either all at once, like drinking a glass of milk, or, more typically, by a constant drip using a pump.

Many formulas are commercially available to use in feeding tubes. Formulas vary in composition, providing different amounts of calories and different types and proportions of carbohydrates, protein, and fat. Formulas also provide various amounts of other nutrients, including vitamins, trace elements (such as iron and zinc), and minerals (such as calcium).

The protein content is often a major difference between formulas. Some formulas have protein that is whole, just like eating regular food or milk. Other formulas have *predigested* protein. Predigested proteins are easier to digest and stimulate the immune system less. There are also formulas made of amino acids (the building blocks of proteins) and other nutrients that are easily absorbed, and these require minimal digestion. The formula may also contain other food substances, such as omega-3 fatty acids, glutamine, or fiber, that some doctors believe help patients who have IBD.

Complications of tubes are usually minor:

- The skin can be irritated by the tape or, in the case of gastrostomy or jejunostomy tubes, leakage of acid or other intestinal fluids.
- Sometimes the tubes, especially the NG or NJ tubes, do not stay

in a good position. This can lead to discomfort, nausea, vomiting, or chest or stomach pains.

- Diarrhea can occur, depending on the type of formula in use.

Less common problems include abnormal blood tests (electrolyte or other chemical imbalances) and aspiration—inhaling food into the lungs (possibly due to vomiting).

Parenteral Nutrition Support

Parenteral nutrition support is nutrition provided intravenously (through the vein). Enteral nutrition support costs less and has less-severe complications than parenteral nutrition, so enteral nutrition support is preferable to parenteral nutrition support. Occasionally, however, a child requires parenteral nutrition support.

Intravenous nutrition may be complete (total parenteral nutrition, or TPN) or supplemental. If it is supplemental, it adds to enteral nutrition or to normal eating by mouth. Although parenteral nutrition usually starts in the hospital, many children are able to go home and lead normal lives (including participation in swimming and most other sports) while receiving parenteral nutrition support. Many home care companies are available throughout the world to assist children and their families with this treatment.

Parenteral nutrition is used for children whose intestinal system will not allow them to absorb or take in all the nutrients they need. Examples include

- children before or after surgery
- children who are severely malnourished
- children whose disease is complicated by
    fistula or fistulas
    short bowel syndrome
    toxic mega colon (a dangerously enlarged colon)
    intestinal obstruction (blockage) or perforation (hole)

Some children receive parenteral nutrition as part of treatment for Crohn disease (see below).

A catheter (tube) that leads into a vein provides parenteral nutrition. The vein may be a small vein (for example, in the arm), or it may be a large central vein (for example, the vena cava, near the heart; figure 13.2). Central veins must be used when long-term parenteral nutrition is given. This type of nutrition is often given at night by pump, while the child is asleep.

Parenteral nutrition requires a special sterile solution. The solution contains calories (from glucose and fat), protein, and other nutrients such as vitamins, minerals, and trace elements (table 13.2). These nutrients maintain health, including children's normal growth and development. Parenteral nutrition solutions can also include some medications (such as antacid medicines).

Complications of parenteral nutrition can be serious, so doctors select patients very carefully for this treatment. Before sending patients home, doctors must make sure that children, parents, and other caregivers receive proper training in the procedures involved with parenteral nutrition.

Complications of TPN can include

- an infection that enters the bloodstream (bactericidal or sepsis), which is the most serious complication
- blood clot (*thrombosis*) of the blood vessel where the catheter is located
- problems due to unusual fluid losses (such as severe diarrhea)
- glucose imbalances (high blood sugar or low blood sugar)

Monitoring Enteral and Parenteral Nutrition

Proper monitoring of enteral and parenteral nutrition support is essential to make sure that treatment is effective. Monitoring also ensures that the treatment is helping to achieve the goals that were set when the feedings started. In addition, monitoring prevents problems from occurring or getting worse.

Parents and other caregivers must watch the child for symptoms or signs of problems, to try to avoid complications. For example, any fever, persistent diarrhea, or vomiting should trigger a call to the doc-

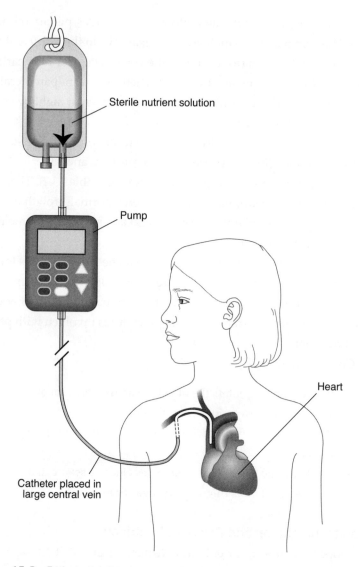

Figure 13.2. Catheter delivering parenteral nutrition. Rarely, children with Crohn or colitis may be unable to eat, and they then require nutrition given by vein. In that case special sterile bags of nutrients may be delivered by pump into a large vein near the heart.

Table 13.2. Composition of parenteral nutrition solutions

Nutrients

Water
Carbohydrate (glucose)
Fat (soybean/safflower oil)
Protein (simple amino acids)
Minerals: sodium, potassium, chloride, acetate, phosphorus, calcium, magnesium
Vitamins: all thirteen known vitamins (A, thiamine, riboflavin, niacin, pyridoxine, folate, cobalamine [B12], pantothenate, biotin, C, D, E, K)
Trace elements: zinc, copper, manganese, chromium, selenium

Other (optional)

Antiacid medications
Insulin
Heparin
Other medications

tor, and your child should be seen in the office or in the emergency room. The health care team always monitors growth and disease activity in children with IBD, but they pay special attention to these factors when children receive special nutritional support.

Disease-Specific Nutrition Considerations

Ulcerative Colitis

Enteral or parenteral nutrition support by itself is not an effective treatment for a child with ulcerative colitis. Treatment in these children relies on medicine or surgery, while the nutritional treatment is usually a supplement for support. Often the nutrition support starts while a child is in the hospital for a serious flare of colitis. In addition to intravenous fluid, corticosteroids, and maybe antibiotics, an enteral feeding tube is sometimes added to supplement eating. Alternatively, and often because an intravenous line is already in place, parenteral nutrition support is used in this situation. Either way, the nutrition is given only to support the child while the medical treatment is taking effect. Sometimes the child also receives nutrition support before surgery to improve wound healing. (Wound healing is sometimes impaired in a child with a poor nutritional state.)

Crohn Disease

Drug treatment is one of the only approaches to improving the symptoms of Crohn disease. Using specialized liquid nutritional formulas as the only source of nutrition for periods of six to eight weeks can reduce intestinal inflammation and digestive symptoms in some children with this disease. Remission rates comparable to prednisone have been reported with formulas. Some studies have also found that children who receive ongoing formula may have fewer relapses.

Formula diets appear to work better in newly diagnosed patients with disease of the ileum (end of the small intestine) than in those who have extensive disease elsewhere or in those in relapse (having a flare). Because of limited data, the long-term benefit of diet treatment over drug treatment is unclear.

The major advantage of parenteral and enteral nutrition, as opposed to corticosteroids, is that the child has less exposure to prednisone. Prednisone will inhibit growth and cause bone weakness, both of which are complications that can cause long-term problems.

Nutrition support can also treat fistulas and obstructions, although these complications often recur when the treatment stops. If the complications recur, then treatment with medications, surgery, or both are preferable to nutritional treatment.

For a child to make normal gains in weight and growth, disease activity must be controlled, and nutritional intake must be adequate for a long time—until the growth of the skeleton is complete. Over the course of the disease, children may need many changes in treatment, including medications, feeding support, and bowel surgery.

Helpful Web Links Regarding Bone Health in Children

National Bone Health Campaign
www.cdc.gov/nutrition/everyone/basics/vitamins/calcium.html

National Osteoporosis Foundation
www.nof.org

NIH Osteoporosis and Related Bone Diseases
www.osteo.org

NICHD Milk Matters Campaign
www.nichd.nih.gov/milk/milk.cfm

Part IV

Living with IBD

ℰ 14
Family Life

A child's chronic illness affects the whole family, and each family member influences the child with IBD. This chapter discusses concerns of parents and siblings of the children with IBD that have been identified in focus group research. (Focus group research involves extensive interviews of many people by professional researchers who attempt to identify what these people have in common. In this case, researchers interviewed families who had a child with a chronic disease.) The chapter also looks at the family as a whole and discusses what we know about what helps families cope effectively when a child has a chronic illness. (Chapter 15 offers insight into how children cope with chronic disease at different stages of development.)

Parents' Concerns

In focus group research, the concern mentioned most often by parents involves how IBD will affect their child's future. Will their child be able to participate in sports and the social activities that are so important to teenagers? Will the child's growth rate and entrance into puberty catch up to his friends? What will happen if she goes away to college? How will he manage dating and finding a significant other? What about having children of her own? Will IBD affect career opportunities?

As adults, parents can see the possible broader implications of having IBD. The unknown is always difficult, but it may be reassuring to know that according to research, people with IBD typically have the same levels of educational and occupational success as the general population.

Young children do not have the capacity to understand long-term implications of their condition. They are more concerned with the immediate future (today or tomorrow). When children are unsure about a situation, they often look to their parents to determine how they should react. As a parent, you can communicate important information about IBD to young children in a matter-of-fact manner, using simple terms. Keeping a straightforward "This is tough but we can handle it" attitude will help your child maintain this attitude, too. Don't worry if your child seems more concerned about day-to-day activities rather than about any long-term difficulties associated with having IBD. This is normal behavior for young children and does not mean that your child has a problem in accepting the facts of the disease.

As children reach the teen years, they begin to understand the possible broader, long-term implications of having IBD, and they may express concerns they have not mentioned before. Follow your child's cues when it comes to answering questions, giving advice, or simply listening and sympathizing. You may want to suggest that your teen discuss these issues with her doctor, with or without you in the room. Your teen would also benefit from getting to know other teens with IBD. As with the young child, the matter-of-fact "This is tough but we can handle it" attitude goes a long way in helping your teen cope with IBD.

Another concern often mentioned by parents in focus groups involves school issues. These issues may include bathroom access, make-up work when the child is absent, taking medications at school, educating school personnel about IBD, and concerns about classmates' and school personnel's sensitivity to the child's needs (see chapter 17).

Additional concerns identified in focus group research include side effects of medications (see chapter 10) and struggling with feelings of guilt. Did I give my child IBD? Why didn't I take her stomachaches more seriously sooner? Am I a good parent?

Many of the symptoms of IBD are not specific and could occur in any number of health conditions. Therefore, there is often a delay in diagnosis. Some research suggests that children experience IBD symptoms for an average of ten months before given a diagnosis of IBD. Even pediatric gastroenterologists, who specialize in children's digestive diseases, don't assume that their own child's abdominal pain and diarrhea means he or she has IBD.

All parents struggle with concerns about being a good parent. Parents of children with special needs (such as a chronic illness) may struggle with these concerns more than the typical parent does. Research has shown that children do best with parents who balance nurturing with appropriate expectations about behavior (and discipline), regardless of whether the child has a chronic illness. There is a wide range of good parenting behaviors, and what you do in the long run, consistently, is most important. Having a child with IBD means that you may face challenges that other parents do not, but otherwise, parenting a child with IBD is no different from parenting any other child.

Siblings' Concerns

In focus group research, the primary concern of siblings was feeling like they were kept in the dark about IBD. Prior to diagnosis, they may have known their brother or sister was ill, but they may have not been told about doctor visits and procedures. Many siblings are taught about IBD during the initial diagnosis and education phase but are less informed about the later course of their sibling's disease. Siblings want to know this information, and they usually have practical questions about IBD: Is it contagious? Is it fatal? Does it hurt? What kinds of medicine will my brother or sister have to take? For how long?

In addition, siblings are often put in the role of a reporter, as family friends and school personnel ask them about their sibling with IBD. Parents can make sure all of their children have the information they need and give them examples of things they can tell others who ask about their sibling.

Siblings may also feel that the child with IBD is favored or receives more of their parents' attention. They may view clinic visits as special times with mom or dad, especially if mom and dad combine clinic visits with a fun activity such as going out to eat. These concerns can be addressed in two ways. First, parents can engage in special, one-on-one activities with each child, not just with the child with IBD. Children love one-on-one attention from parents. Activities can include playing board games, helping with cooking, riding bikes together, reading aloud together, or working on a special project.

Second, parents should require all children, including the child with IBD, to follow all the usual family rules, live up to the same expectations, and share the same level of responsibility. The child with IBD can be expected to join in family recreational activities and to have the usual responsibilities and chores. Do not avoid disciplining the child with IBD, if discipline is necessary. Allowing a child with IBD to avoid responsibilities and discipline deprives the child of opportunities to learn how to cope with life—and with having IBD in the context of normal family life. It may also create problems with siblings, who may feel that the child with IBD is favored.

Family Concerns

Some families seem to take IBD and its challenges in stride. How do they do it? Researchers in other pediatric chronic illnesses have identified what helps families cope effectively. These families balance the demands of the illness with other family needs and responsibilities. Family life does not revolve around the illness. The illness must play a large role at times, but family life does not regularly center on it. These families also have clear family boundaries and expectations. They maintain their usual family routines. They require all children, including the child with IBD, to follow all the usual family rules, live up to the same expectations, and share the same level of responsibility, as well as receive consequences for inappropriate behavior.

Successful families have supportive social networks. Support systems, both formal and informal, can provide both ongoing emotional support and the periodic practical support needed in managing clinic visits and hospitalizations. Such practical support may include transporting other children to and from school and activities. These families also have flexible family roles that can change as needed, and an open communication style that allows all family members to express feelings and needs.

In successful families, all family members, including siblings, have knowledge about the symptoms, treatment, and course of IBD. Fi-

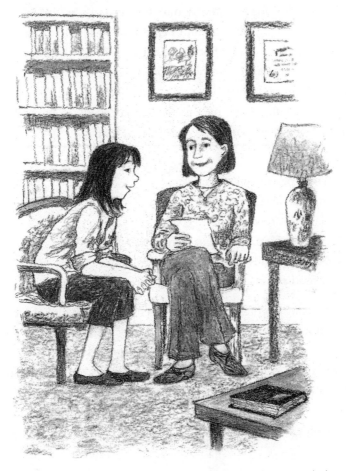

Talking with a counselor, psychologist, or social worker may help control stress or anxiety in a child who has a chronic illness.

nally, successful families use active coping strategies. Active coping strategies include problem solving and actively seeking social support. Passive coping strategies include denial, avoidance, and withdrawal.

When to Seek Help

Since IBD affects the whole family, and since each family member affects the child with IBD, it is important to recognize when counseling would be helpful for any family member. Therapy with a psychologist, psychiatrist, or other mental health professional is a good idea any time behavioral or emotional problems significantly interfere with a person's performance in any area, such as school, work, social activities, or family relationships.

Specific warning signs of a problem that needs to be addressed with professional help include

- lowered grades
- lowered productivity at work
- significant absences (from school or work)
- social withdrawal
- lack of pleasure in social or recreational activities
- significant family stress in addition to IBD
- increased arguments with spouse, parents, or siblings

Mental health professionals who specialize in health psychology can help the child with IBD and other family members cope with the disease as well as its consequences. Taking medications on schedule, managing pain, feeling distress about medical procedures, and avoiding school—these and other stresses are often managed better with the help of a professional who can offer support as well as advice about practical things the child and family can do to help everyone cope.

✵ 15
Different Ages,
Different Issues

Living with inflammatory bowel disease is not easy. It is a chronic condition, with unpredictable flareups of symptoms that are difficult to manage. The symptoms include abdominal pain, bloody diarrhea, and low energy. In addition to the flareups, long-term problems related to IBD include malnutrition, slow growth, and late puberty.

IBD may have an unpredictable course. Patients may undergo invasive tests, complicated treatments, and sometimes surgery. All of this means that a diagnosis of IBD can be difficult to accept, particularly during childhood and adolescence. Most children and teens go through a period of adjusting, both in their emotions and in their behavior, to a diagnosis of IBD. Many children experience periods of anger and even depression.

Several factors influence how a person reacts to having a chronic illness. How your child responds to IBD depends in part on his age, his maturity level regarding cognition (thought processes), and the severity of the illness. Another factor in a child's reaction to the diagnosis is the parents' reaction. Parent-child conversations about IBD are essential, and they usually set the tone for the whole family. This chapter discusses developmental landmarks—the differences in maturity and coping styles of children at different ages. This information will guide parents who are helping their child or teenager cope with IBD. Talking to your child in an age-appropriate and matter-of-fact way will help your child cope with IBD and everything that goes along with having this disease. Our goal is to help you help your child live a fulfilling, productive life despite having a chronic illness.

Early Childhood: Ages 2 through 6

A child with IBD faces special issues that are connected to his developmental needs. Between 2 and 6 years of age, a child has many physical, emotional, and cognitive targets to reach. By reaching these targets, the child develops the independence, self-control, and language skills needed to begin school successfully.

Physically, the healthy preschooler grows more slowly than a baby. Parents notice that their child has less of an appetite than he had as an infant. A preschooler's eating habits can change noticeably from day to day. It can be difficult to tell the difference between normal appetite changes at this age and a reduced appetite from worsening IBD. Watch your child's growth carefully to make sure that the IBD is under control. Your child's doctor may need to order tests to help determine if IBD is making your child's appetite worse.

During early childhood, the main developmental work of the child includes

- improving self-control (for example, toilet training)
- learning a language
- getting used to separating from parents or other main caregivers

During the preschool years, language skills advance rapidly. Your child's vocabulary is growing noticeably, and sentences are more organized and complex. Preschoolers are also better at expressing their feelings and needs. Although children at this age may sound more adult, they see the world very differently from adults. For example, they are afraid of monsters, or they have imaginary friends. It is normal for preschool children to express feelings of stress through behavior instead of words. Preschoolers are also fascinated with their bowel functioning.

In terms of cognitive growth, children in this age group often show both real-world, concrete thinking (everything happens because of something I can see or touch) and magical thinking. Magical thinking means thinking that events in their lives happen because of their own thoughts, feelings, and behaviors; magical thinking also means mixing up cause and effect. While this view of the world is normal preschool behavior, it also affects how your child reacts to having IBD. Children may connect the symptoms of their disease with unrelated events or actions. Young children diagnosed with IBD often connect their symptoms (such as pain and diarrhea) with other events that happen at around the same time. For example, a 5-year-old may think that her bad behavior caused her IBD, and she may feel guilty.

The preschooler's "magical" view of the world can create challenges for her and for her parents when it is time for treatments or tests. Young children may have mistaken ideas about the reasons for procedures or hospitalizations. It is not uncommon for them to see such activities as a form of punishment rather than as being necessary for their care. In addition, they have difficulty understanding ideas such as amount and length of time (for example, "it will last only a short while" or "this will hurt only a little"). Parents often want to explain, "You need to have this blood test so the doctor can make you feel better." An explanation like this is usually not comforting at this age and can even add to the child's worry. The company of a calm, comforting parent is most important to the preschooler. Most children's hospitals have child-life specialists who can help children prepare for procedures, and they have a wealth of advice for parents.

Preschoolers often have a good idea of outside body parts, but inside body parts are still not real to them, and children connect them with many magical ideas.

Preschoolers worry about loss and about being left behind. These anxieties can complicate their reactions to medical stresses. They may be sad and angry about being separated from siblings during hospitalizations, or they may feel jealous about the good health of siblings, especially if the preschooler does not have the physical energy to take part in regular activities. Preschoolers who feel overwhelmed may behave like babies again (this is called *regression*), or they may lose skills they already learned (for example, toilet training).

You can help your young child with a new diagnosis of IBD by encouraging him to talk about the illness and by answering your child's questions in simple language that the child understands. Listen for elements of magical thinking that may be making your child nervous. Expect reactions such as "forgetting" about his illness during times of remission (when the disease is not active), or not showing distress even during IBD symptom flareups. These reactions can be considered normal as long as your child cooperates with medical care and reaches all the right developmental landmarks. Watch your child for changes in behavior or play. If you are concerned about your child's feelings, talk about your concerns with your child's pediatrician or pediatric gastroenterologist. They may have suggestions. It is often helpful to consult a mental health professional who specializes in helping children and parents adjust and cope.

Parents need to manage their own anxiety about the diagnosis and treatments of IBD. If you do not have a good support system, you need to put one in place. Talking things over with other adults, and knowing you can call on them for logistical assistance if you need to, will help you be available for your child. Finally, as mentioned in the previous chapter, it is critical to keep daily family life as normal as possible, including discipline. Your child needs to develop a self-image well beyond "being sick." Instead, your child should think of IBD as one of life's manageable challenges.

Middle Childhood: Ages 6 through 12

In middle childhood, children try hard to master their bodies and the environment. As children enter school, they become more independent and are more concerned about being accepted by their peers. Self-esteem is an important issue. In the child's mind, how she does in school, sports, and play are measures of how much she is "worth." She tries to master skills such as school behavior, sports, and special talents. A diagnosis of IBD can interfere with the physical energy a child needs to do well in school and follow other pursuits and can negatively affect a child's self-esteem. With the diagnosis of IBD, the apparent loss of control (for example, rectal bleeding, bowel movement accidents, and invasive procedures) challenges the child's need for mastery and skill development. This apparent loss of control can cause anxiety and feelings of helplessness. Children may also be fearful about falling behind in school, and their fear or actual lagging behind may make them feel isolated from others their age.

Children may choose not to perform certain activities that might show they are "different" because of their IBD. Feeding tubes or central venous catheters (devices for easy vein access) can be a big source of insecurity for children. At a time when children are having their first sleepovers, even taking medication in front of friends can be embarrassing. Not being able to go to school because the disease is active can distance children from friends. They may feel overwhelmed and unable to catch up when they are ready to return.

Children of this age still use real-world, concrete thinking, and they may also still have unusual beliefs about why they are sick or why they need to go to the hospital (for example, the hospital is a punishment). As they mature, they begin to understand difficult information about how the gastrointestinal system works, though they may still have mistaken ideas about what causes problems. A child may understand that he is having abdominal pain because the IBD is irritating his intestines but may still secretly believe it is because of an unrelated event, such as being unkind to his sibling. Discuss these feelings with your child. Understanding your child's worries can help you encourage him to overcome them. Finding and encouraging his strengths can improve self-esteem.

School-age children may become more and more focused on the effects of the treatments on their bodies and may begin to display fears of bodily harm and death. Middle-school-age children tend to focus on the present. Because of this, it is best to tell them about procedures no more than one week ahead. This will help them handle the situation best and decrease the possibility of intense negative reactions.

Ask your child questions to make sure he understands the facts about IBD and its treatment. Let your child know it is acceptable to have negative feelings about the diagnosis, such as fear, frustration, and anger. Many children in this age group will express their feelings, ideas, and fantasies about IBD through play, such as drawing or role-play—they may play doctor, for example. Encourage your child's use of these methods to help him cope with IBD-related stresses, such as medication, IVs, or injections. Use techniques such as distraction and relaxation to help him express his feelings during procedures.

Educating your child's friends and their parents about your child's IBD can help create a supportive environment. Excusing your child from the normal responsibilities that his peers and siblings have (homework, picking up, clearing the table, and other chores) can send him a harmful message. It can make the child's fear and worry worse, or the child may begin to use symptoms to avoid doing unpleasant tasks. Your expectations of your child need to be reasonable, taking into account your child's health. If you have questions about appropriate expectations, talk with your child's pediatrician or pediatric gastroenterologist.

IBD can present challenges that are too difficult for families to face alone. In these instances, outside help is a key to success. Making regular visits to your pediatrician or pediatric gastroenterologist help make sure that the disease is under control and that your child is growing well. Other specialists may become important members of your child's health care team, too:

- Dieticians or nutritionists can help with your child's nutrition and, as a result, their growth.
- Psychologists can help patients and families cope with the emotional challenges of IBD.
- Child-life specialists can help the family prepare for stressful procedures and cope with hospitalizations.
- Physical and occupational therapists can help your child get back to her best possible activity level after a period of serious illness.
- The school nurse and your child's teachers can help ensure the

best educational environment for your child; talk with them about your child's IBD so that they understand your family's needs.

Your pediatrician or pediatric gastroenterologist can help you identify and contact these specialists.

Adolescence: Ages 13 through 18

Adolescence (the teen years) is the exciting transition from childhood to adulthood, beginning with puberty in early adolescence (12 to 14 years old) and ending with late adolescence (17 to 19 years old). This is a time of physical, emotional, and cognitive maturation, often with maturation in these different areas developing at different rates.

Adolescents begin to move from concrete thinking (thinking in terms of what is real or what exists) to abstract thought (having theories about the world around them). Adolescents tend to think more about their actions and the reasons they act in a certain way. The teenager's main task is to develop a sense of self-identity in order to move successfully from the family world to the outside adult world. Teenagers are very concerned with being accepted by their friends—their friends' approval is more important to teens than their family's approval.

The rapid physical changes associated with puberty produce sharp self-awareness as well as concern about appearance. Poor growth or delayed sexual maturation, which many teens with IBD have compared with their healthy peers, can make concerns about appearance worse. Medical procedures that involve loss of function can be particularly difficult (a colostomy, for example). Accepting authority and giving up control to their medical team can lead teens to feel helpless and dependent. These are particularly difficult feelings in this age group. For all these reasons, adolescents with IBD may become challenging or rebellious when it comes to medical treatments, in an effort to regain a sense of control.

Teens have a growing understanding of the complicated causes of IBD, both environmental and genetic. This new awareness may increase fears about the possible long-term effects of IBD and its treatments. At this stage, concerns about what the disease might mean for the rest of the teen's life increase. Teens with chronic illnesses are likely to overstate the possible restrictions that come with their condition (for instance, "I'll never be able to play sports"). Or they may choose to participate in risky behavior (such as smoking) to be accepted by their friends.

Most people with inflammatory bowel disease believe that stress can make the symptoms of their disease worse, and accumulating medical evidence shows that they are right. There is no doubt that IBD causes stress for teens, their parents, and their siblings. Even without symptoms of active disease, the teenager often worries about whether the symptoms will come back and prevent them from going on a school field trip, being on the basketball team, or going to the senior prom.

The stress is greater when teens have symptoms of active disease. They worry about making multiple trips to the bathroom while trying to attend school, or about how the medicine they take will change the way they look. An even bigger stress occurs during the complete disruption of their life due to surgery or a stay in the hospital.

Parents are often stressed by the competing demands of a career and caring for an ill child. Siblings are also affected. They are concerned about their brother or sister's health, and they often feel left out. They feel that they are not always told what is happening and that talks affecting their lives take place without them (see chapter 14).

When a teenager's lifestyle and activities are affected by the symptoms of IBD, or by worry and depression related to the disease, the problem must be recognized. Such reactions are normal and appropriate, and your teen needs support. Support groups are often helpful for adults with IBD, but less so for teenagers. If they feel well and have no symptoms, teens would rather think the disease does not exist, ignore it, and not talk about it. If they have symptoms that they cannot ignore

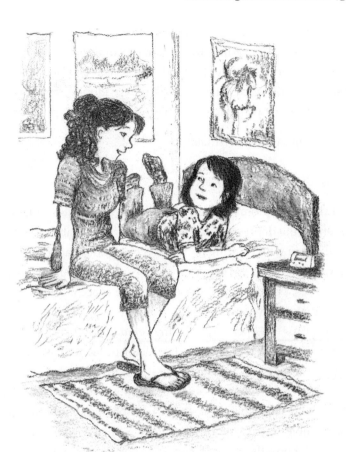

Siblings often rely on each other for support. When a child has a chronic illness, it is important to educate other family members.

(though they may try), they often do not want their friends to know about it, and they do not want to talk about it with their peers.

More than most chronic diseases, IBD can have a very strong effect on the life of a teen. With encouragement, trust, and respect for privacy, teenagers will express their anger and frustration about their disease. They can do so with adult family members, an adult friend, or their doctor. When they do talk about it, they should be shown ways to cope and to minimize the interruption in their life. Sometimes learning coping skills from a professional counselor is helpful.

The teen years are an important developmental period, when young people learn to adjust their emotions in ways that work best in different situations. Although mood swings can be normal, teens diagnosed with IBD appear to be at risk for developing serious depression. Parents must watch for early warning signs of depression:

- constant sadness or irritability
- changes in sleep habits
- loss of interest in fun activities

Report these symptoms to your child's doctor so that evaluation and treatment of the depression can start as early as possible.

For the teen who is trying hard to develop independence, maintain privacy, and gain acceptance from his peers, IBD is an embarrassing and, at times, humiliating disease. It can be especially difficult for a teen to discuss bowel habits and to tolerate invasive physical exams and tests. Thus, an open and trusting relationship between the teenager and his doctor is essential. The doctor needs to trust her patient to tell her, when asked, what is going on in the patient's life and what symptoms he has. Teenagers deserve to know that their doctor will tell them the truth about their disease and not hold back information. They should be able to trust that their doctor will answer questions completely and honestly. Furthermore, in most situations, the doctor's physical exam and conversation with the teenager should be done privately. Separate time should be set aside for discussion with the teenager, the parents, and the doctor together. The teen should always be part of discussions regarding major changes in the treatment plan.

Older teenagers insist on more independence and begin thinking about life after high school, including living away from home. They should slowly be given more responsibility for their own health. One example of increased responsibility is letting teens be in charge of taking their medicines. Although they should remember to take their own medications, parents should still check on them. Checking can be done by refilling the teen's prescriptions or checking the weekly pill minder. If teens are refilling their own prescriptions, parents should check to make sure prescriptions are refilled on time.

Doctors can also give older teenagers direct access to them, by offering them their business card with phone numbers and e-mail address. Although many teenagers do not use it, they do carry the card or keep it at home. The card is a powerful reminder of their independence, and of their doctor's trust in them.

The severity of IBD is not always related to the severity of the disease's effect on a teenager's life. Both parts—the severity of the disease and effects of the disease—must be recognized and addressed by everyone involved in the teen's life. By promoting independence, you can help your teen develop self-confidence and a sense of being able to take care of herself, even in the face of a chronic, challenging illness like IBD. In this way, teens with IBD can reach their full potential as adults.

Late Adolescence and Young Adulthood: Ages 18 through 21

All young adults face a challenge when they begin to consider what they will do after high school, be it going to college, getting a job, or moving away from home. Many consider distance from home and family to be a major part of their decision. Young adults with IBD also face the challenge of leaving behind health care providers and family members who have been their support system while living with IBD.

Young adults need to know that their goals and hopes for the future come first. For example, a young person may want very much to attend a university that is clear across the country from where they have been receiving medical care, because the school offers exactly what they are looking for. She should be encouraged to attend that school regardless of her IBD. Her physician should make every effort to identify a doctor who cares for IBD patients in her college's location. If a young person has no interest in going to college or leaving home, IBD should not be her excuse in making that decision.

Fortunately, young adults have more mature coping skills than children do, and they are able to handle the consequences of IBD better, but naturally they feel apprehensive about how IBD might affect their ability to perform at school or at work. If they experience health-

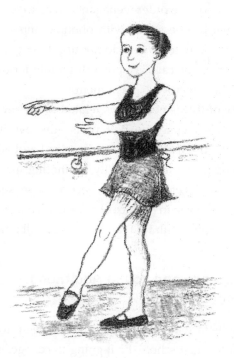

related problems at school or at work, they deserve support and encouragement. They may also want to consider modifying their schedule. A few careers may not be possible for someone with IBD (as is true with any other chronic disease), but luckily those careers are few.

Many teenagers and young adults believe that IBD interferes with dating. Young adults start to wonder how IBD may affect their long-term relationships and their chances of becoming parents. They may worry about this issue even though they do not intend to start a family in the near future. Their doctor can give them reassuring information.

IBD undoubtedly interferes with the lives of people of all ages, and it affects their family and friends as well. For some, IBD can be easy to ignore. For others, it is a major inconvenience and can be a disabling disease. Nevertheless, IBD should not and need not prevent anyone from setting and achieving goals in sports, leisure activities, education, career, and family. Children, adolescents, and young adults are able to cope better and have more reasonable expectations when they are given encouragement, support, and accurate information.

Parents and caregivers play a critical role in helping their child cope with and accept an IBD diagnosis as easily as possible. The following guidelines can be helpful for parents and caregivers of children of all ages:

- Be open and honest, and use language your child understands when discussing the diagnosis of IBD with her.
- Help your child understand that showing feelings is normal and is a part of the learning experience in dealing with a chronic illness.
- Observe your child for constantly extreme emotional or behavioral reactions; if such reactions are present, consider getting support for your child in the form of counseling or support groups.
- View your child as having IBD. Do not let IBD define your child. Observing this distinction will help you support your child's healthy move to adulthood.

Several Web sites devoted to IBD offer content ranging from medical facts to personal stories. As with all Internet use, make sure you are using a Web site that is monitored by responsible individuals or organizations to avoid reading misleading or inaccurate information, whether it is posted deliberately or in ignorance. Recommended Web sites include the IBD Experience Journal (Children's Hospital Boston) at www.experiencejournal.com/ibd, Crohn's and Colitis Foundation of America at www.ccfa.org, North American Society for Pediatric Gastroenterology, Hepatology and Nutrition at www.naspghan.org, UC and Crohn's: A Site for Teens at www.ucandcrohns.org, and IBD U, at www.ibdu.org.

16
Complying with Treatment

Compliance (also called *adherence*) means following the doctor's advice and recommended treatment. It means always taking the medications the doctor prescribed, following the recommended diet, and making any other necessary changes in lifestyle, as recommended by the doctor or other specialist. Compliance is a major concern for professionals who care for patients with chronic illnesses such as IBD.

Studies have shown that when a doctor recommends a plan or prescribes a medication to a patient with a chronic illness, the patient complies only about half the time. There are two main reasons for noncompliance with medical recommendations. The first is that the patient or the family does not agree with the doctor's plan, and the second is that the patient feels worse when he starts taking the medication, so he stops taking it. When the patient or his family members do not share their concern with their doctor, or the doctor doesn't explain the potential side effects of the treatment, problems with compliance can occur.

Young children will need their parents' help in complying with medical treatment. For parents and older children, compliance is easier when they understand *why* they are having a problem adhering to medical advice. If the issues are clear, then the patient, family, and doctor can address the issues together.

If you or your child are not following your doctor's recommendations, consider whether any of the following issues apply:

- Do you and your child understand IBD, including the fact that the disease is long lasting and requires long-term treatment? Do you understand the complications that can occur if the disease is left untreated, or if it does not respond to treatment?

- Has your doctor told you and your child what side effects to expect from the treatment (whether the treatment is medication, diet, or something else)?
- Does good communication and trust exist between the patient, family, and health care provider?
- Are family or social influences causing problems with adherence? One example is a family in which the parents are separated, and the child with IBD spends time in two households.
- Has the family had past experience with health care providers that affects their acceptance of prescribed treatments? Or does the family have cultural beliefs that affect their acceptance of prescribed treatments?
- Is the patient concerned about the stigma of being seen taking medications? Or does the patient have concerns about other visible signs of having the disease (for example, feeding tubes)?
- Is the child's stage of development interfering with compliance? The age of a person with IBD can affect her adherence; teenagers especially, as part of their normal development, may rebel against authority.
- Is the treatment plan very complicated? A complicated treatment plan—medication schedule, difficult-to-follow diet—may cause problems with compliance.

What Can You Do to Ensure Adherence to the Medical Plan?

Your child needs to get the greatest benefit from her medicines and other treatments. The following section offers guidelines to make sure your child and the rest of the family receive all the benefits of the medical advice provided to them.

Education
- You and your child (if she is old enough) should understand her medications. Your doctor can give you information about

what the medications should do, and what possible side effects
they have. When you get the prescription filled, your pharmacist can give you more information.

- If you are worried about the side effects of the medications, talk
  about your concerns with your child's doctor and the IBD team.
- Some side effects are "normal," while others may be a concern,
  so you need to have a good understanding of side effects. Some
  medications have side effects when your child first starts taking
  them, but the side effects may get better as the child's body gets
  used to the medication.

Treatment

- Work with your doctor to come up with a treatment plan that
  your child can adhere to.
- If not being able to sleep is one of the side effects of the medicine, your child may be able to take the medicine in the morning. If being sleepy is a side effect, your child could take the
  medicine at night. Check with your child's doctor or pharmacist to make sure that it is okay to take the medicines at these
  different times.
- It is important to take the medications at regular times every
  day. They work best if the amount of medicine in the blood is
  always the same.
- If you (or your child) are tempted to stop any medication, think
  hard about it first. Some medications take several months
  before they start to work. If your child stops taking them, it
  may be several more months before they work again. Your
  child could get sick during that time, without medication to
  keep his symptoms under control. Do not stop a medication
  without talking to your child's doctor.
- Many medicines keep the symptoms of IBD from returning. If
  giving medications to your child when he feels well seems to
  make no sense to you, remember how your child felt when the
  disease was active.

- If you have trouble remembering when to give your child medicine, try a few tricks:

    Give him his pills at the same time every day.

    Link giving the pills with another activity that your child does at the same time every day, like taking a shower or brushing their teeth.

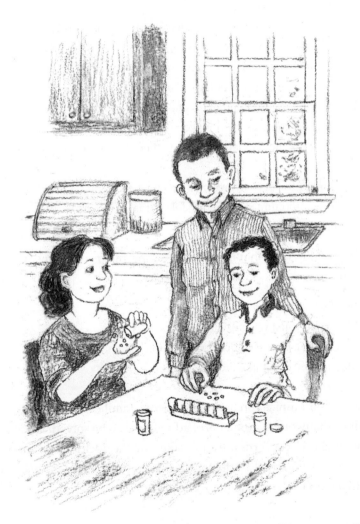

For patients taking many different pills each day, a pill box is a useful aid. Various kinds of pill-reminder boxes can be easily found in most pharmacies.

Put sticky notes in a place where you will see them, like on a
mirror. Change the place of the notes occasionally so that
you do not get used to seeing them and start ignoring
them.

Use a weekly medication dispenser (available at your
pharmacy) to help keep track of whether doses of medication were taken or not.

- Store the medications properly, in sealed, original containers
  with the label intact, and in a cool, dry place—unless the
  medication should be kept in the refrigerator.
- Renew the prescription before it runs out. Don't leave it to the
  last minute. If your child is a teenager and it is his responsibility to renew the prescription, you should still have an understanding that he will let you know when the medication runs
  low.
- Remember to get new prescriptions written at the regular
  doctor's appointment to avoid delays that might cause the
  medicine to run out.

If your child is still having trouble taking his medications, try to
figure out why.

- Maybe taking them is a "hassle."
- Maybe they just wish IBD would go away.
- Maybe they have a difficult medication schedule.
- Maybe they don't like the side effects.

With good communication between patients, families, and health care
providers, many of the problems of adherence can be solved. Find our
what your child's concerns are and make sure the doctor knows about
them, too. Ask your child's doctor to help you and your family come
up with a plan for handling these concerns.

❧ 17

School Days

Going to school to get a good education is an important task of childhood. School is also where much of a child's social and emotional growth occurs. Therefore, with some exceptions, the ability to attend school regularly is an important measure of good health. School provides an education in the whole experience of new expectations, learning to live with schedules, and dealing with teachers, friends, and new challenges. School is also about boyfriends and girlfriends, clubs, lunch hour, the gym, and a lot more.

Children with any chronic disease are at some risk for failing at school. Like all children, children with inflammatory bowel disease find the school experience at times stimulating, boring, scary, and confusing. The emotional highway between the brain and the bowel is never busier than when a child is at school. Even healthy children experience stress from academic and social expectations—stress that can result in symptoms such as nausea, abdominal pain, and diarrhea. Since the connection between the gut and the brain is so strong, it is not surprising that many children with IBD experience uncomfortable symptoms while at school.

When a child is sick, the school experience may be exhausting and overwhelming. As in any chronic disease, however, normal activity is good medicine. Getting to school and seeing friends is a good distraction from symptoms. Keeping busy helps a child work up an appetite and makes a child tired enough so that she can fall asleep at night. This daily rhythm is important to the development of a healthy body and just as important to the medical care of the illness.

Although a child or teenager with IBD may not be able to make it through a full day of school on some occasions, it is still important for her to participate in school activities. Doing so may require some negotiations with teachers or the school principal. We advise parents to reserve home schooling for the worst times of illness, such as during recovery from surgery.

Discuss frequent school absences with the medical team. If your child is missing a lot of school, she needs better medicine or counseling. She may need both.

Better medicine sometimes means stronger medicine. Many people with IBD try to minimize the amount, strength, or number of medicines they take. They feel that taking medicine is a sign of weakness, or that it is not "natural." Most doctors agree that you should take as few medicines as possible when you are well. If you have a medical condition, however, you are better off taking a medication that helps you lead a more normal life, even if the thought of taking medication is worrisome or scary.

If your child has to take medication at school, you can talk to the teachers about the best way to store the medication and how your child can take it with the least disruption to his regular school schedule. Alternatively, your child's IBD doctor or the clinic nurse can make suggestions about how to fit the medication schedule into the school schedule.

Your child's IBD doctor can also help with planning for school trips outside your area. The doctor can create a medication plan that will minimize the chances of a flareup, but it is still a good idea to have an emergency action plan in case of a flare. This emergency plan should include a list of medications to treat a flare and, if possible, the name of a local medical contact, in case problems occur.

There are a few special challenges for kids with IBD at school. For one thing, everyone hates being embarrassed. Some kids are embarrassed because having IBD and taking medication makes them feel different. Others are humiliated if they must request many trips to the bathroom. Sharing the diagnosis with a few close friends is probably the best medicine for this problem. Also, the teacher may agree to allow the child to leave the room unobtrusively if he needs to go to the bathroom.

Most kids find that close friends will come together around them. The child or teen might practice talking to friends beforehand through role-play with his family or counselor. This gives him a chance to find the words he is comfortable using with his friends.

The expectations at school can sometimes become a problem. Teachers are used to hearing excuses all day long. Children in a wheelchair do not have to "make excuses" and explain that they have problems walking, but children with an invisible handicap like IBD sometimes do not get the same consideration. This is where communication becomes so important. Most teachers will try to be helpful if they know the whole story. You or your child's doctor can provide teachers with information. Helpful pamphlets for teachers are available from the Crohn's and Colitis Foundation of America (CCFA). The information can help your child and her teachers set reasonable expectations regarding schoolwork, assignment deadlines, and tests. It can also help to ask for unrestricted bathroom privileges in advance.

Your child may experience particular problems dealing with the bathrooms at school. School bathrooms are rarely supervised, and they can be scary places. It is important that you, a counselor, or the teachers help your child or teenager solve these problems. Solutions include using the staff washroom and carrying a deodorizer spray.

Without a doubt, other issues will come up at school. Many IBD programs have support groups, either ones that meet face-to-face or ones that exist on the Internet. You may find that your child with IBD has a lot in common with children who have different illnesses. The ability to problem solve with other children of the same age can help your child find solutions that make her feel more comfortable at school and at home. The process of helping someone else with her problems is one of the more effective ways for a child with a chronic condition to adjust to her own condition and grow stronger.

Growing up involves taking chances, but it is mostly about learning to make good choices. School offers children, especially those with a chronic illness, many opportunities to make hard choices and learn from them. Some studies found that kids with IBD are stronger, more mature, and have better self-esteem than kids without serious diseases. Repeatedly making hard choices is like physical conditioning. "Reps" make the child or teen stronger.

❧ 18

Insurance and Other Financial Issues

Both Crohn disease and ulcerative colitis are conditions that require long-term medical follow-up and treatment. The costs of care greatly vary depending on the disease severity. Patients with mild disease may have affordable medical expenses, but patients with severe disease will experience considerable expense. Many of the new medications are very expensive; for example, one year of infliximab infusions can cost over twenty thousand dollars. In addition, some patients with both Crohn disease and ulcerative colitis may require hospitalizations and more intensive treatment. Because people with IBD are likely to accrue high medical costs, health insurance is essential.

In the United States, employers provide many different types of health insurance policies. The policies vary significantly, with some providing only catastrophic coverage (they only go into effect for a prolonged hospitalization), and others providing comprehensive outpatient and inpatient coverage. In general, if a family has a member with IBD, the family should if at all possible obtain a comprehensive insurance policy with a low copay for outpatient visits and a generous drug benefit plan. This way, if a child requires an expensive medication, it is more likely to be covered by insurance.

Because of the expense of many of the newer medications (infliximab, adalimumab, certolizumab), many insurers review the medical plan after the physician prescribes the medication. A nurse reviewer or physician at the insurance company will ask the physician to fill out a form with pertinent aspects of the patient's history (this is called a prior authorization form). Based on the medical information the company receives, they will either approve or deny the physician's prescription. A denial is not always permanent; it often means that the insurance company requires additional information about the patient's medical condition before it considers paying for a very expensive drug. Such information may include the patient's diagnosis; what other therapies have been tried in the past; published medical evidence that the prescribed drug is effective; and alternative treatments to be considered.

If the physician provides all this information and the insurance company continues to deny the claim, then an alternative approach may need to be taken. In such cases, an attorney or patient advocate may be useful. One nonprofit organization that specializes in obtaining needed health care for patients is Advocacy for Patients with Chronic Illness (www.advocacyforpatients.org)

As a child with IBD becomes a young adult, he also must be aware of the need to keep health insurance. While most children can stay on their parents' plan while they are in college, they usually must find their own plan after graduation. Depending on their parents' insurance plan, young adults who are full-time students can often stay on their parents' policy until age 23 (or sometimes 25). The types of health insurance plans offered by an employer may be one factor in determining where the young adult chooses to work (see chapter 19).

Family and Medical Leave

Although most children with inflammatory bowel disease are healthy and can participate in all school and extracurricular activities, at times the illness may require extra parental attention and involvement. This is particularly true in children with more severe forms of Crohn disease and colitis, or children undergoing surgery. In some cases, a parent may need to take time from work to care for his ill child. In the United States, the Family Medical Leave Act (FMLA) allows parents to formally request *unpaid* leave from their employers for up to twelve weeks in a year to care for an immediate family member with a serious health condition. Requirements to be eligible for FMLA include working for the same employer for at least twelve months and working for a company that employs at least fifty people. Although FMLA does not provide pay for family members who choose to take time from work, it does protect employees from being fired because they are caring for a sick relative. To apply for FMLA leave, both the employee (parent) and the child's physician must complete paperwork documenting the nature of the child's medical condition.

Disability Benefits

Most patients with IBD lead healthy lives or have mild symptoms and therefore are not eligible for disability. Under rare circumstances, however, a child's or young adult's IBD may be so severe that she may be eligible for disability benefits (Supplemental Security Income, or SSI). Being approved for SSI may allow a child to be eligible for Medicaid benefits. Applying for SSI is a long and difficult process that usually requires the assistance of an attorney. Careful documentation of "marked and severe functional limitations that are expected to last at least 12 months" is required. Such limitations may include severe anemia, malabsorption, malnutrition, obstruction, or abdominal abscess.

The regulations regarding insurance coverage and patient's rights change rapidly, and it is possible that by the time this book is published, different federal or state regulations will be in place. What's important is that parents and patients know that both federal and state regulations are in place to protect families with chronic illness. Excellent resources for families who have questions relating to financial concerns, insurance coverage, and employee leave include the following:

- social workers at your hospital
- attorneys who specialize in disability and medical insurance
- the Crohn's and Colitis Foundation Web site: www.ccfa.org
- the Advocacy for Patients Web site: www.advocacyforpatients.org

Part V

As a Child Grows Up

ℰ 19

Transitions from School to Work and Independent Living

Children growing up with a chronic illness such as inflammatory bowel disease face even more challenges than other children their age. This chapter highlights some of the more common physical and emotional problems faced by a child with IBD during some of life's normal transitions.

Transition to Middle School

Many physical and emotional changes and challenges accompany the transition from elementary school to middle school.

Physical Development and Puberty

As with other chronic conditions, IBD may cause a delay in puberty. Children with IBD may be smaller than all their friends. Girls may not start their periods or have breast development when their friends do. These delays are not usually a cause for long-term concern. Children with IBD should be reassured that even if they enter puberty later than their friends do, they will eventually catch up. All children need information about the physical changes that will happen to them during puberty. Let your child know that these changes are part of the natural process of growing into adulthood.

A number of factors influence the timing of puberty (sexual maturation):

- family traits
- hormones—the chemicals in the body that cause puberty
- nutrition factors or weight issues
- disease activity and the location of your child's disease

Delays in puberty can be the result of malnutrition, not getting enough calories in the diet, or malabsorption (when our bodies cannot take in the vitamins and nutrients they need from the food we eat).

In girls, the first sign of puberty is usually breast budding, which starts on average at the age of ten years, but it can happen as late as age thirteen. Menstruation (getting a period) usually starts about two years after the start of puberty. You should talk to your daughter's healthcare provider if she has no puberty-related changes by age thirteen, or if she does not get her period by age fifteen.

Boys normally enter puberty one year later than girls do. The first signs are enlargement of the testes and thinning and reddening of the scrotum (the sac containing the testes). These signs usually occur at age eleven, but in children with IBD, they may be delayed until age fourteen, or even later.

Steady growth during middle childhood results in height increases of about two inches per year in girls and boys. Weight increases on average by approximately six pounds per year. One of the first signs of IBD may be a short build, especially if the child has Crohn disease involving the last part of the small bowel. If the disease has been under good control for several months, and the child is not growing in height, you should talk with the doctor. The doctor might recommend testing for other disorders (for example, thyroid disease, celiac disease, or diabetes).

Nutrition

Good nutrition is very important for a young person's overall health and well-being. A varied and balanced diet supports growth, energy, and general health. For best growth, your child should be eating a diet high in calories. The diet must also be rich in calcium to support bone growth and strength. A low-fiber, low-residue diet is recommended only if narrowing is present in the bowel (low-residue diets leave very little material in the bowel). Talking with a dietician about the best diet for your child's particular needs can be helpful.

While certain foods might make the symptoms of IBD worse in some people, there are no specific foods that your child should avoid. No evidence shows that inflammation of the intestines is affected by the food a person eats. Middle school, however, is a common time for lactose (milk sugar) intolerance to appear. Inability to break down the sugar in milk and other dairy products can lead to gas, bloating, abdominal pain, cramps, and diarrhea. An easy, noninvasive test known as a lactose breath test can diagnose this condition. An over-the-counter dietary supplement containing the enzyme lactase, which breaks down milk sugar, is available to take with dairy products to prevent symptoms.

Coping with the Stress of Illness in Middle School

Children with inflammatory bowel disease often have more stress in their daily lives than others their age. For example, they must cope with taking medications daily (or multiple times per day), frequent doctor visits or hospitalizations, painful examinations, injections or blood draws, body-image issues related to delayed growth and puberty, and sometimes surgery. Although no one can avoid stress completely, the following suggestions may make things a little easier:

- Always inform your child of what lies ahead concerning medical tests and treatments. A child's worry is often due to fear of the unknown.
- Listen to your child and encourage him to express emotions, whether he is sad, frustrated, angry, or fearful. Be supportive and always try to listen to what he is *not* saying (in other words, try to read between the lines).
- Talk openly about the illness so your child feels comfortable with the topic.

- Talking to other children who have gone through the same or similar experiences can be valuable. Your child may relate well to other children with inflammatory bowel disease. It often helps your child to realize that he is not the only one with this condition. Other children with IBD (and perhaps their parents) may be able to share helpful coping strategies for home and school.

- Focus on your child's strengths and talents. A child with IBD often feels discouraged. Many children with IBD are also angry about the restrictions placed on physical activity, or about the discomfort of the disease. Many children derive great pleasure and pride from various creative activities such as playing a musical instrument, drawing, painting, or writing. A hobby such as collecting coins, stamps, or baseball cards can also be fun and instill feelings of success. In addition, academic success should always be encouraged and rewarded. Like adults, all children need to feel a sense of accomplishment.

- Encourage your child to begin to take an active role in his health care (if he doesn't already). Allow him to participate in the decision-making process whenever possible. For example, allow your child to pick which arm to use for a blood draw and to decide whether he wants a numbing cream before a test. Also, allow for some flexibility in scheduling an endoscopic procedure or x-rays so that the child can weigh in on the decision. If a bowel preparation is needed prior to the tests, give the middle school child some options. Options will help your child follow the bowel preparation procedures more willingly and give him a sense of control.

School Issues for the Child with Inflammatory Bowel Disease

During the middle school years, children want to look and behave like their peers and participate in the same activities. They want acceptance from their classmates, possibly more than at any other time in their school years. They shape their self-esteem and self-image by this acceptance.

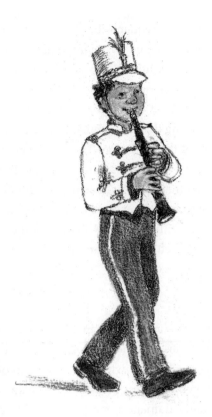

Keep teachers informed and updated regarding changes in your child's medical condition. For example, if your child's appearance has changed, meet with your child's teachers before the child returns to school. Teacher meetings are the key to preventing unnecessary problems in your child's progress at school. Children spend most of their time in school, and teachers may be the first to notice a flareup of the disease. They can let you know about changes in behavior, lack of attention, and signs of depression or anxiety. Teachers can also tell you how your child interacts with classmates, and they will keep you updated on academic performance.

Relationships with Peers

IBD can present a special challenge for children as they relate to their age group. Any condition that requires medications, specialized bathroom privileges, or frequent absences from school can result in embarrassment. When helped by their friends, family, teachers, and healthcare professionals, children can develop into stronger individuals, overcoming many barriers.

Some parents urge their children to hide their illness and medications from peers, fearing that their child might have to endure ridicule if others are aware of the condition. This may send a wrong message to the child, telling her that IBD is a shameful condition. Instead, children should be encouraged to disclose the condition to close contacts in a comfortable setting. Telling close friends can greatly ease the isolation many children with IBD feel. A teacher or the school nurse may be helpful in guiding children through the process of telling their friends about their illness.

Sports

Children with IBD should participate in sports if they want to. Studies show that bones become stronger and denser when physical activity is increased. Children with IBD should avoid spending too much free time watching TV or playing video games. These inactive hobbies may actually damage bone growth and add to decreased bone density (resulting in weaker bones). Coaches, parents, teachers, and health care providers should be supportive of a child's athletic activities. In return, the child with IBD should do his part by taking prescribed medications, eating a balanced diet, drinking plenty of fluids, and getting plenty of rest.

Transition to College Away from Home

Many young people with inflammatory bowel disease find the adjustment to college to be more complex than they expected because of health issues they need to deal with. Being away at college is often the first time in a young adult's life that she is managing her own health without a parent's daily assistance. There are new routines, and sometimes no routines. Finding the college that is the best fit is a challenge for everyone, so a student with IBD needs to realize that her illness should be only one among many factors she considers while choosing a college. A young adult with IBD is more than a patient, and if she is unhappy with her choice of school, health and studies often suffer.

IBD should not preclude exploring academic institutions away from home. The decision to attend college far from home or as a commuting student is an individual one. Still students with IBD should anticipate some considerations to help make their transition to college as seamless as possible while they maintain the continuity of their health care.

Preparations

As soon as a college or university has been selected and the student has been accepted, contact the school's Dean of Students with Disabilities Office or Disability Support Office. This helps establish with the school that it might need to make accommodations for the student with IBD so that if the student needs to make future or unpredictable requests, he has less work to do in the moment of medical need. This is also the office to use for residential accommodations, including requests for

- a private bathroom
- a private room
- permission for a refrigerator in the dorm room
- permission for a car on campus (if appropriate)

Many students with IBD had Section 504 plans in high school that provided academic accommodations so that their studies were not compromised. Section 504 plans are written agreements between parents and schools that provide reasonable accommodations for children with disabilities. For a child with IBD, a 504 plan may also outline a disease management plan. College authorities can often help the student develop similar plans to provide accommodations in schedule or housing in the college environment. Revising the high school 504 plan so that it is relevant to the particular school's curriculum is usually done through the disabilities office or the dean of students, and this should be initiated as soon as possible.

Before the student heads off to college, he should find out what services are provided by the university health clinic: labs, pharmacies, radiology services. For the student on maintenance medications, it is helpful to scout out where prescriptions can be filled when on campus. Many families have drug plans that provide Internet access to pharmacies that directly ship medications to students living out of town. If this service is not available, traveling to college with at least a month's supply of daily medications is a good idea because it allows time to set up with a new pharmacy and have prescriptions transferred to be filled locally.

For students not attending school close to home, plans should be made to identify a gastroenterologist near the school campus. Students may still see their primary gastroenterologist at scheduled visits or may decide it is time to transfer care. Either way, it is important to have a physician close by in the event of sudden illness. An initial appointment should be scheduled as soon as possible after arriving on campus so that the new gastroenterologist can review the student's complete history, medication schedule, and test results.

Lifestyle Considerations

Once on campus, the new student with IBD will have much to consider. Many patients have certain foods in their diet that cause symptoms or flareups. Parents need to be realistic about their children's college eating habits; there will always be leftover dinner for breakfast and vice versa. It is the student's responsibility to make attempts to eat correctly and to maintain a nutritious diet.

Often, the dietician at the campus dining halls can provide guidance on menus at the various campus or dorm locations as well as options that can easily be made available as standing alternatives to meal plans. Patients receiving nutritional supplements may want to identify a primary dining hall for use and ask the disability support services to keep some supplements in the cafeteria refrigerator for easy access without the student having to return to the dorm.

College can also demand the development of new strategies and creative ways for the student with IBD to maintain a healthy lifestyle. Once on campus, it may be helpful to make note of the locations of campus bathroom facilities, both inside and outside academic buildings, as well as the hours they remain open. Remembering to take medications can be more difficult with new schedules and many more distractions. In this high tech age, reminders can come in many forms: cell phone alarms, watch alarms, pop-up reminders on a laptop or wireless technology; low-tech also works—sticky notes or taping medicine bottles to the mirror.

College campuses provide many opportunities for students to engage in risk-taking behavior. Such behavior is an even bigger gamble for students with chronic illness than it is for other students. Exposure to and use of alcohol and recreational drugs are dangerous in general but can be especially harmful to students with IBD. A student with IBD not only faces all the common risks, but also must consider how these substances interact with her prescribed medications and that they may trigger a flareup.

Disclosure: Who Should I Tell?

A common concern of students with IBD heading off to college is determining who to talk to about their IBD. Staff of the student health service should always know about a student's medical history. Whether others should know, however, is a personal and private issue.

The student does not have to tell anybody about his IBD, but finding and sharing the diagnosis with someone he can trust and who can provide support if a medical complication presents itself, especially if the student is away from home, is an important consideration. Many students decide to seek out and confide in and rely on other students with IBD or another chronic medical condition.

The decision about how much to share and with whom should be guided by personal priorities and comfort level. Many students initially choose to tell only their roommate, and eventually they share the diagnosis with close friends. Often, it is also helpful to alert academic advisors or academic mentors, especially if questions arise about lighter schedules or curriculum selections.

The student at first may not know anyone who has medical issues such as IBD. Universities draw a wide array of students, however, and many students have medical issues they must contend with in addition to their academic studies. The college environment is now more accepting of the needs of students and even values the diversity that differences bring.

Checklist

In an effort to ease the transition to college and reduce additional stress amid an already significant life change, we created the following quick reference list of the things your student should consider as she leaves home for college:

Medical Care
- ✓ Do I have all the vaccinations I need? Are they up to date?
- ✓ Who should I contact if I am not feeling well?
- ✓ How should I contact these identified individuals: by phone, e-mail, via parents?
- ✓ What are the important phone numbers and e-mail addresses to take to school to allow easy contact with family members or physicians?
- ✓ How can medical team members best return my calls? What is the best route for the medical team to contact me: by voice-mail, e-mail, pager, phone, my parents?
- ✓ What health services are available on campus?
- ✓ Has a local gastroenterologist near campus been identified?
- ✓ How can I schedule an introductory appointment in advance of a necessary appointment?
- ✓ Have copies of medical records been sent to the local doctor and university health services in advance?

✓ Where can I get blood draws and laboratory tests done?

✓ What is the fax number of the local laboratory?

✓ To whom and to what fax number or address should a local lab send test results?

Medications

✓ How much of an initial supply of medications should I bring to campus?

✓ Where can I store medications?

✓ Should I inform roommate(s) of my medication schedule and medical needs? How will I explain this?

✓ What are the steps to take to avoid running out of medications, and what can I do if this still occurs?

✓ What is the address and phone and fax numbers of the local pharmacy?

✓ What are the requirements for sending prescriptions in advance to my new pharmacy?

✓ What is the most convenient and accessible avenue to keep medications refilled: local pharmacy or mail-order pharmacy?

Diet

✓ Can I tolerate the dining hall food?

✓ Will I have regular access to sufficient and adequate calories?

✓ Should I bring supplements to campus?

✓ Are there relevant food restrictions? Are there foods I cannot eat?

✓ How does alcohol interact with my IBD medication(s)?

Housing

✓ What will be the setting: dormitory, apartment, house?

✓ Will I have roommates?

✓ How accessible and private are the residential toilets?

✓ Where are the bathrooms located around campus?

Transitioning to college is exciting and scary at the same time, for student and for parents. There are many responsibilities, and even more possibilities, for the young adult heading to college. The healthier your child is, the more she can enjoy this exciting time and take advantage of all the opportunities that college can provide.

Transition to Work

Health Insurance Considerations

One of the most important issues that young adults with IBD must handle as they enter the work force is maintaining health insurance coverage. Young adults who are full-time students can often stay on their parents' policy until age 23 (or sometimes 25), depending on their parents' insurance plan. When a young adult is no longer a student, however, or reaches the maximum age covered by the policy, he can no longer be covered under his parent's insurance.

As health insurance is no longer an automatic benefit of employment in many circumstances, the employee must pay close attention to the benefits offered by his new employer. Because transitioning from school to the work force usually involves the simultaneous transfer of health coverage from the family's plan to an employer's policy, the newly employed person with IBD must explore different potential employers' health insurance policies. It is also necessary to compare the various coverage choices that may be offered by a single employer, including HMOs, PPOs, point of service (POS) plans, or fee-for-service plans.

When combing through the plans' options, consider

- frequency of visits covered
- number of visits covered within a calendar year
- flexibility and ability to choose specialists not only for IBD but also for associated problems, such as arthritis (rheumatologists), nutrition (dieticians), and coping (mental health professionals)

Take care to examine the fees associated with maintenance out-patient visits, emergency room visits, lab work, x-rays, in-patient hospital stays, and mental health coverage. The fees for these services should be balanced against the employee's cost of the plan and the flexibility the plan offers in choosing preferred providers. While an HMO may be more affordable, the time spent obtaining referrals from a primary care physician for various subspecialty providers is often not worth the physical cost of prolonging access to necessary care, especially when such care will be a recurrent need.

Because IBD is a chronic illness, one of the most critical considerations when transferring from a previous policy to a new employer's policy is that not more than sixty days elapse without coverage before the new policy becomes effective. If an employee has a gap in health insurance coverage for more than sixty days, the new policy has the right to decline coverage of any routine, maintenance, or emergency care related to a preexisting condition—such as IBD. If there is less than a sixty-day gap before the new policy takes effect, the new policy must cover the costs associated with any preexisting condition, including IBD.

The sixty-day rule is noteworthy because many employers' policies do not become effective immediately upon employment. Therefore, the employee must take care to make sure there is no gap between the termination of an old policy and the commencement of a new one. *Often, a young person entering the workforce must purchase additional months on a parent's health plan through COBRA (the Consolidated Omnibus Budget Reconciliation Act), or have a discussion with a potential employer's human resources director about appealing the standard date of effective coverage through a company's plan.*

Many young adults with IBD simply choose not to consider interviewing at agencies or companies that do not offer health insurance. People living with IBD have the benefit of *knowing* they have a chronic illness that can force unpredictable demands on their lives. Using that information to make an informed decision allows the job seeker to be proactive in identifying options for reasonable coverage. If an ideal job opportunity does not offer adequate health insurance, a person has the option of purchasing private policies through major insurance carriers. These can be costly, but they are often less costly than a large hospital bill or the physical cost of not getting adequate maintenance care and suffering a potentially preventable flareup.

Disclosure to Employer and Co-workers

A new or potential employee has no legal obligation to disclose any personal or health-related information to her employer if her situation does not substantially interfere with work responsibilities or performance. It is not necessary to tell a prospective employer about an IBD diagnosis during an interview. The interview is an occasion for an employer to assess a candidate's fit for the position based on skills. It is a time for a candidate to learn about the position, its associated responsibilities, and the resources and benefits available on the job so that she can determine if it fits her needs and goals.

Once the employee starts a new job, she faces new personal and professional challenges. One such personal challenge is deciding with whom and when to share personal facts. Outside the performance of work, all other aspects of one's life are personal, and personal information is shared with co-workers at the discretion of the employee. When a person has a condition such as IBD, however, it is necessary to consider how to best manage medical and employment responsibilities. If the symptoms of IBD act up, who among one's colleagues would be most affected? How might supervisors react? Would they be more understanding if they had the knowledge that IBD symptoms were affecting an employee's ability to work, or would they use the knowledge maliciously?

It is important to identify people who can be trusted and share the diagnosis when the time seems right. In many circumstances, telling an immediate supervisor before the employee necessarily feels comfortable telling peers or co-workers may be appropriate. Should IBD symptoms flare, or an unpredictable and urgent complication arise, it may be helpful if an immediate supervisor is aware that the employee has a condition that remits and relapses. Her understanding of the nature of IBD can minimize employment problems before they occur. It may, for example, prevent your employer from interpreting a last-minute absence from work soon after beginning a new job as reflecting a poor work ethic.

Assessing the Work Environment

With any potential job, make sure there is realistic and reasonable access to health care. While a person with IBD should not compromise his career goals, it is practical to consider the degree to which a particular job might make it difficult to obtain necessary healthcare in a timely manner. For example, a young adult patient with IBD had always looked forward to working on a cruise ship so that he could travel and see different parts of the country and world. This lifestyle clearly posed barriers to the continuity of health care. To reconcile this goal with the reality of knowing that his IBD required frequent attention, he applied only to major cruise ship lines with established health insurance plans, and he deliberately requested certain itineraries that docked at ports in major domestic and international cities. These cities had well-established medical centers.

IBD doesn't have to rule out jobs requiring work abroad. Most developed countries have physicians who can provide appropriate care if medical demands arise. Take the experience of another young adult patient who had always dreamed of doing missionary work. Rather than abandon this goal because of her IBD, she consulted with her gastroenterologist and selected assignments in areas of the world with developed medical centers that she could easily reach in case of emergency.

The physical environment of a job is also an important consideration, including accessibility to bathrooms. For instance, does a job opportunity require frequent travel? If so, is this in a car or via airplanes? Would being on the road frequently lead to anxiety about access to bathrooms? Would it hinder optimal quality of life and success at work?

Reviewing environmental stressors and potential triggers of symptom flares is important when considering a new job. Some jobs may take place in a setting where there is a lot of cigarette smoking, something that might provoke an IBD attack. Working in a restaurant or bar, an employee might be more likely to eat the establishment's food, which in a person with IBD might encourage a diet that disagrees with his digestive system. In some industries and jobs, having a drink with a client is a large part of the culture, but such an activity might at times be difficult for someone with IBD. Therefore, being aware of what triggers your disease and how environmental factors stress your body and personal course of IBD can influence your career choices. These factors do not necessarily mean a job should not be pursued or accepted; however, for many individuals, these are practical issues to consider when IBD is part of daily life.

Choosing the Best Fit and Finding a New Routine

Ultimately, young adults should not design goals and career aspirations around their IBD. However, it is often necessary to reconcile the demands of IBD with career choices. How flexible is a workday? Does the company offer compensation time ("comp time," in which hours missed from work are made up at another time) for doctors' appointments, or does it require employees to use vacation or sick time for medical needs? If so, would this become a disincentive to taking the time to care for your health? If a person is out of work beyond a certain number of days, is she required to use short-term disability and receive lower pay?

Young adults with IBD need to rely on practical self-assessment and sensible self-monitoring, since it is often not clear how IBD might be affected by the demands of work. Work commitments can be even more erratic or demanding than those experienced in high school or college. As the job becomes familiar, it is often helpful to build in some sort of predictability so that the known demands of IBD can be incorporated into the workday. This can mean finding new times of day to take medications, or new places to keep a duplicate supply of medicine, so that a last-minute out-of-town meeting or the need to work exceptionally late for a deadline does not prevent access to maintenance medications. It can also mean packing a lunch or keeping select foods available in the office refrigerator to avoid dietary triggers. Reconciling issues such as these with your personal course of IBD will help you transition successfully into the workplace.

20

Transitions from Pediatric to Adult Health Care Providers

The vast majority of children with IBD in the United States receive their IBD-related medical care from pediatric gastroenterologists. When the children become young adults, however, they usually outgrow their pediatric gastroenterologist and transition to an adult gastroenterologist. Such transitions are often challenging because the patient and the physician have become close over the years, and separation is difficult. In some countries, the transition from a pediatric to an adult GI practice is very sudden, occurring on schedule when a child turns a certain age. In the United States the transition often happens as children are either entering or graduating college (or reaching college age) and is done when the patient and the pediatric physician mutually agree that the time for transition has arrived. Thus, the patient has time both to mature and to prepare for the transition.

In addition to leaving a physician they are familiar with, patients transitioning from pediatric to adult GI practices may find they are leaving a *system* they are familiar with, too. The many differences between pediatric and adult GI systems in the United States are summarized in table 20.1. The primary difference between a pediatric and an adult system is the health care provider's expectations of the patient. In a pediatrician's office, the parents attend every visit and often provide most of the patient history. For a child with a chronic illness, it is not uncommon for that pattern of parental input to persist in the pediatrician's office even after a child is mature and perfectly capable of doing most of her own talking. Once a child becomes a young adult

Table 20.1. Differences between pediatric and adult GI practices

Pediatric	Adult
Often hospital and university based	Often practice based
Multidisciplinary (several specialties in the same office)	Gastroenterologists only
Family focus	Individual focus
Protective, paternalistic	Collaborative
Emphasis on parental responsibility	Emphasis on patient responsibility
Generalistic, social focus	Disease focus

and "graduates" to an adult practice, however, the parents may not even be allowed into the examining room. At this point, patients need to provide a complete history themselves, and take down all the doctor's recommendations and act on them without input from their parents. This may be a challenge for a young person who has been used to mom and dad taking care of things.

Taking Ownership of IBD While Becoming a Young Adult

The transition to the adult-based system is both inevitable and desirable; to help make the transition go smoothly, we recommend a graduated approach. This approach involves preparing the teenager starting in high school to acquire the skill set necessary to be both a "good patient" and an effective advocate for his own medical needs. Some of the skills needed for a successful transition are summarized in table 20.2.

Parents can help in the process. Begin preparing your child in late middle school or high school for more independence and autonomy. Ask him to speak when he goes to the doctor, even if the doctor is looking at you. Over time, make sure the child knows what his diagnosis is (Crohn or colitis), where the disease is located (ileum, colon, etc.), and what medications and doses are prescribed. After a child is in middle to late high school, offer to step out of the room at an appropriate time, so the child and doctor have some "alone time" to-

Table 20.2. Tips for a successful transition to an adult practice

- Begin preparing the adolescent during high school.
- Transfer during or after college (ages 19 to 23).
- Clarify involvement of family members.
- Note milestones and benchmarks indicating the right time for transition. The young adult with IBD
    - is knowledgeable about the diagnosis and what it means
    - knows the location of her disease
    - understands his medications
    - has a psychosocial support network
    - books her own appointments
    - carries his insurance information

gether. This alone time serves two purposes: it enables the child to gain a sense of independence, and it allows the doctor to ask sensitive questions. During the child's later teenage years, the physician will be an important source of counseling about high-risk behaviors (sexual activity, smoking, alcohol) that should not be discussed in front of the parents because it is important for the child to feel free to speak honestly and to ask the physician questions.

After a child turns 18, she is legally an adult and entitled to autonomy. At that point, the parent should discuss with the young adult patient whether the patient wants the parent in the room during the visit. In addition, the physician may ask the patient for permission to disclose medical information to the parents. At this point, it is the patient, not the parents, who determines the degree of information sharing and involvement. Most patients, however, continue to rely on their parents as trusted advisors and welcome participation in the visits. Once the patient transitions to an adult practice, however, parents will probably need to stay outside the clinic room and learn about the details of the visit from their child.

In addition to the challenge of transitioning from a pediatric to an adult care delivery system, the young adult may also be required to change health insurance policies. In the United States, children are typically covered by their parents' health care policy through college. When the child enters the work force, however, she must find (and pay for) her own insurance. In a child with inflammatory bowel disease, finding the proper policy is essential. Some patients with IBD, especially those receiving biologic therapies, may have drug expenses that are over twenty thousand dollars per year. If insurance does not cover the expenses, they are at risk of disability. Therefore, a young adult with IBD entering the labor force must carefully look at what health coverage an employer offers before choosing a job. Larger companies and universities generally offer better coverage than small companies, which offer better coverage than self-employed individuals. Although there is currently a national political discussion about a universal health care system in the United States, it is unclear at the time this chapter is being written whether such a system will be implemented. At this time, a young adult with IBD needs to factor health insurance into career and life decisions.

In conclusion, the journey from childhood to adulthood is frightening for some individuals and exhilarating for others. Parents and physicians must support the transition to independence and empower the patient to gain ever increasing amounts of responsibility. If a young adult is neglecting his health (for example, missing appointments, not taking medications, or not keeping health insurance), parents and providers need to encourage the patient to get back on track. At this vulnerable age, peer and patient support groups, such as those offered by the Crohn's and Colitis Foundation of America, may be invaluable.

Part VI

Additional Information

❦ 21

Complementary and Alternative Medicine

While conventional medical therapy for Crohn disease and ulcerative colitis has greatly improved over the last twenty-five years, it is still far from perfect. Medications commonly used to treat IBD may have unpleasant side effects for some people. In addition, many of our most effective medications (immunomodulators and biologics) reduce the activity of the immune system and therefore may increase the risk of infection or lymphoma. Nutritional therapy, while safe, often requires patients to stop eating and to drink formulas that don't taste very good. Because IBD is a serious illness, because we don't have perfect treatments, and because there is no cure at the present time, many patients investigate complementary and alternative medicine (CAM). The United States National Institutes of Health defines CAM therapies as "a group of diverse medical and health care systems, practices, and products that are not presently considered to be part of conventional medicine." CAM treatments include dietary supplements, megadose vitamins, massage therapy, acupuncture, magnet therapy, meditation, yoga, energy-based therapies such as therapeutic touch, and spiritual healing. While standard medical approaches go through a long and careful research process to prove they are safe and effective, CAM therapies do not, so information about the effectiveness of CAM treatments is less reliable.

Surveys taken over the past several years showed that about half of children and adults with inflammatory bowel disease seek CAM treatments. CAM treatments for IBD include acupuncture, dietary supplements, diet, and relaxation therapy. Most likely, those who seek CAM treatments represent a portion of patients who are not responding well to conventional treatments. Few studies exist to determine the effectiveness and safety of CAM treatments for IBD, and physicians generally do not receive formal training in the use of CAM. Therefore, physicians sometimes do not discuss CAM treatments with their patients. Many patients hear about such therapies from friends or read about them on the Internet. To date, there is not enough evidence to recommend CAM therapies routinely. Nevertheless, this chapter will review some of the complementary treatments used for IBD.

Acupuncture

Acupuncture, one of the most important medical practices in traditional Chinese medicine, has been used for thousands of years. Though acupuncture came from China, it is now practiced routinely in many Asian countries, including Japan and Korea. Acupuncture has been used to treat numerous symptoms, including chronic pain, nausea, and motion sickness, as well as inflammatory conditions like inflammatory bowel disease. Surveys demonstrate that many patients with IBD get acupuncture treatments, and some small medical studies suggest that acupuncture can help patients with IBD.

Acupuncture is based on the principle that everyone's body has channels of energy running through it. These channels are called *meridians*. The energy is called *qi*, or *chi*. According to traditional Chinese medicine, disease occurs when the energy in the channels is disrupted or imbalanced. Stimulating the appropriate meridians can help regulate the flow of qi and correct any imbalances. In acupuncture, this stimulation is accomplished by inserting very fine needles along certain points. The points are areas where the meridians come to the skin surface. These same acupuncture points are used in other disciplines, including Shiatsu massage and acupressure.

It is still unclear exactly how and why acupuncture works, but there are many theories. The most accepted theories involve possible effects on the nervous system and the circulatory (blood) system. Acupuncture may affect the nervous system by causing the body to release substances called *endorphins*. Endorphins are pain-relieving substances that act like the pain medicine morphine. They are thought to be the substances responsible for the runner's high that marathon runners get after running or training for long periods. The release of endorphins would, in theory, provide relief from chronic pain.

It is also possible that acupuncture causes nerve cells to change how they communicate with each other. It may accomplish this by changing levels of *neurotransmitters* (chemicals that turn nerve cells on and off). Acupuncture may also prevent pain signals from being transmitted to the brain. This theory is based on the assumption that nerve fibers can carry only so many signals at a given time. If having acupuncture can stimulate a given nerve path enough, the path may be unable to carry pain signals at the same time.

Acupuncture may also cause small blood vessels running near the skin to relax, which increases blood flow. This increased blood flow could potentially have an effect on healing or regeneration of the tissues of the body. Increased blood flow could also affect the immune system by carrying immune cells to and from certain sites.

When performed correctly, acupuncture should not hurt. Some people notice a tingling or similar feeling when the needles are inserted. Sometimes the needles are twirled, heated, or attached to low electrical currents to help with the stimulation of the meridians, which may cause some sensation during the acupuncture session. Acupuncture should always be performed with sterile needles, which are often disposable and used only one time. Following an acupuncture treatment, some people feel lightheaded or dizzy, and it is appropriate to plan for someone else to drive them home after a session.

Some people may find that acupuncture works well for certain symptoms associated with IBD, such as nausea, abdominal pains, or joint pains, but it may not work for other symptoms, such as diarrhea or blood in the stool. Using acupuncture as a form of treatment for IBD should always be done under the guidance of an IBD physician.

If acupuncture is done correctly, there is little risk in receiving an acupuncture treatment. However, there is risk to any treatment if it is used incorrectly or as a replacement for another treatment that is known to work. There is no reason, based on what we know about acupuncture, to stop other IBD treatments in order to have a good response to acupuncture. If acupuncture is considered as a treatment for IBD, it should be seen as a "match" that goes together with Western medicine therapy, rather than an option that replaces Western medicine therapy.

Alternative Nutritional Therapies

Fish Oil

Some early studies found beneficial results in people with IBD who took large amounts (2.7 to 5 grams/day) of omega-3 fatty acids, found in certain fish. This form of fish oil, predominantly eicosapentaenoic acid (EPA), decreases formation of inflammatory cells and chemicals of inflammation. Fish oils have been shown to have an anti-inflammatory benefit in some adults with heart disease. There have been two controlled studies in Crohn disease; the initial study from Italy suggested it might be helpful, but a larger study from Canada has not shown any effect. There is little information about fish oils in ulcerative colitis. Diarrhea has been reported as a side effect in some studies.

Short-Chain Fatty Acids

Bacteria in the colon convert unabsorbed carbohydrate, protein, and fiber into short-chain fatty acids (SCFAs), hydrogen, and carbon dioxide. The SCFAs are important for normal function of the colon. SCFA levels are decreased in severe ulcerative colitis, so studies have been done to test the effectiveness of SCFAs (given by enema) as a treatment for patients with ulcerative colitis. To date, none of these treatments has shown benefit.

Probiotics

Probiotics (good bacteria) may provide some benefits to health. Probiotic compounds are made of bacteria that populate the intestinal tract and generally do not cause disease. *Lactobacillus* and *Bifidobacterium* species are commonly used in probiotic treatment. A number of probiotic preparations are available in supermarkets, health food stores, and over the Internet. Probiotics may reduce intestinal inflammation by decreasing the activity of the immune system. Studies in infants and young children suggest that probiotics given at an early age may reduce the severity of viral diarrhea, antibiotic-associated diarrhea, and allergic disease.

The role of probiotics in Crohn disease and ulcerative colitis remains a topic of active research and interest. Several studies of probiotics in the treatment of Crohn disease have not demonstrated any benefit. In ulcerative colitis, many small studies have suggested a possible benefit. One area where probiotics might be of use is in pouchitis (inflammation in the pouch made by the surgeon from part of the small intestine following removal of the colon; see chapter 11). Studies of a probiotic combination called VSL3 (a mixture of eight different bacterial species) suggest that the probiotic may reduce symptoms of diarrhea in pouchitis.

In summary, probiotics offer a safe and potentially effective complementary therapy for IBD. Determining which probiotics are safe and effective, however, and what the best dose is requires further research. More studies would help our understanding of the role probiotics play in treating patients with IBD.

Antioxidants

Early evidence suggests that oxidative damage plays a role in triggering inflammatory bowel disease. Oxidative damage is damage caused to DNA and other parts of the cells. The cause of this damage is a chemical reaction involving materials that take electrons from other materials in the cells. Levels of vitamin E, selenium, and vitamin C (all antioxidants—they protect against oxidative damage) were found to be low in a small number of people with IBD. Studies are needed to determine the role of taking supplementary doses of these and other antioxidants (such as vitamin A) in inflammatory bowel disease.

Special Diets

As discussed in chapter 13, nutritional therapy has a significant role in the treatment of IBD, particularly in children with Crohn disease. To date, however, no one diet has been scientifically proven to maintain remission in inflammatory bowel disease. Two diets that have achieved some popularity as complementary therapies in the IBD patient community are the Specific Carbohydrate Diet and the Maker's Diet.

The Specific Carbohydrate Diet (SCD) was developed by Elaine Gottschall, a nutritionist who hypothesized that restricting the intake of processed foods (particularly carbohydrates) could lead to alterations in the intestinal bacteria, which could in turn help maintain remission in IBD. The diet has also been tried in a number of other conditions, such as autism. Foods not allowed include processed meats and most forms of starches and sugars. This diet is quite rigorous and challenging to follow, especially in a teenager. It is also unclear if and when benefits are seen, though some patients do claim it improves their symptoms. Additional information on this diet can be found on the Web site www.breakingtheviciouscycle.info. The Maker's Diet, popularized by Jordan Rubin, is a diet similar in many ways to the SCD; it too relies on restriction of simple and complex carbohydrates. The diet also emphasizes fresh fruits, fresh vegetables, and home-made foods, including sprouted wheat or spelt bread.

These diets are difficult to implement, they are expensive, and their effectiveness is unclear. Because they have not been carefully studied, they are not routinely recommended by physicians. If a parent is interested in trying this therapy, they should discuss it with their doctor to review the risks and benefits.

CAM for Managing of Chronic Pain

Pain is a common symptom in people with inflammatory bowel disease. In most patients, pain can be controlled by reducing the bowel inflammation with medical or surgical therapy. In a few children and adults, however, pain is a persistent problem. In people with IBD and chronic pain, the physician must perform a thorough evaluation (possibly even repeating x-rays, upper endoscopy, or colonoscopy) to make sure the IBD is being adequately treated. This is particularly true in children with Crohn disease, where narrowed areas of bowel may cause symptoms of cramping due to obstruction (blockage). In addition, the physician must consider other organs in the abdomen that might cause pain: the pancreas (pancreatitis), liver (hepatitis), gallbladder (cholecystitis), kidneys (kidney stones, urinary tract infection), and bladder (cystitis).

In a large number of patients, a thorough medical evaluation fails to identify a specific cause of pain. Pains that occur in the absence of identifiable bowel inflammation are often termed *functional pain*. These pains are not imaginary. They often occur because even after inflammation has been successfully treated, the bowel may remain sensitive, or irritable. Treatment of functional pain is complex, and a detailed discussion is beyond the scope of this book. Patients with functional pain may benefit from treatment with various medications, including gabapentin and amitriptyline. In addition, hypnosis, acupuncture, relaxation techniques (to reduce stress), and counseling are often helpful in treating such pain.

ℰ 22

Where to Get Additional Help and Information

If your child has just been diagnosed with inflammatory bowel disease, or if you or your child have had the disease for a number of years but have some new questions, where do you go for information? Ideally, at the time of diagnosis you were given information on IBD. Some hospitals routinely provide newly diagnosed IBD patients with an information packet. Print brochures published by the Crohn's and Colitis Foundation of America (CCFA) are probably available in your gastroenterologist's office. If they are not, ask your physician to order some, or call your local chapter of the CCFA.

If you were not given any information, or if you have additional questions, the Internet is a quick and easy source of information. Typing "inflammatory bowel disease" into an Internet search engine will result in hundreds of thousands of pages you can visit. But there are problems and pitfalls in such searches. The first problem is the enormous amount of information you can find. The second is that these sites cannot be used as a reliable source of information when it comes to *your* care or that of your child. The information on the sites is often based on general information, or on one person's experience. This experience may or may not be related to you and your disease. So how do you begin to sort through this overwhelming amount of information? How do you know which information is right for you or your child?

Happily, there are several very good sources of information on the Internet. Even if you do not have Internet access at home, you can get access at school, at work, at your friends' houses, or at the public library.

One of the first sites you should visit is the Web site of the North American Society for Pediatric Gastroenterology, Hepatology and Nutrition, at www.naspghan.org, which is a valuable resource for patients and parents of children with IBD. Among its other benefits, it allows parents to search for NASPGHAN-affiliated pediatric gastroenterologists (children's digestive disease specialists) in their area. In addition, there are informational brochures in English, Spanish, French, and Portuguese.

NASPGHAN and the Children's Digestive Health and Nutrition Foundation (CDHNF) cosponsor a Web site made specifically for children with IBD, their parents, and their health care providers. The site can be found at www.kidsibd.org. This site contains selected links to IBD information.

Another early stop on the Internet should be the Crohn's and Colitis Foundation of America, at www.ccfa.org. This is a comprehensive site for inflammatory bowel disease. CCFA has reliable and up-to-date information. In addition to disease information, this Web site features webcasts on important topics, such as an eating-out guide for people with IBD. You can also find information about CCFA chapters in your area. If you join a CCFA chapter, you will receive newsletters and information on various activities, which may include support group sessions, IBD camps, and fundraisers. While most of the information on CCFA.org is for adults, this Web site also contains information for children with IBD. The CCFA site has links to other important sites that may be helpful, including information about clinical trials. The CCFA also has a print comic book aimed at children ages 7 to 14 called *Pete Learns about Crohn's and Colitis*, which can be ordered from the Web site.

Another Web site, www.ucandcrohns.org, is cosponsored by CCFA and the Starlight Children's Foundation. This new site is aimed at adolescents with IBD. It features information and videos written and spoken in a language that is clear and appropriate for this age group. A sister Web site, www.ibdu.org, provides information for patients with IBD who are headed to college.

Another interesting, informative, and well-organized site is the National Institutes of Health (NIH) site at www.nlm.nih.gov. On this site, search for "inflammatory bowel disease." This NIH site has links to the latest news on Crohn disease and ulcerative colitis as well as information in Spanish and an interactive tutorial. There is information on the anatomy of the digestive tract, and you can view a colonoscopy. The site has a link to government-sponsored clinical trials and information on pamphlets published by the CCFA and other organizations, such as the American Gastrointestinal Association. The site includes relevant laws and policies, as well as information for children and teens.

Other helpful Web sites include

- Reach Out For Youth with Ileitis and Colitis: www.reachout foryouth.org
- The J-Pouch Group: www.j-pouch.org (This site has information specifically for people who are considering a colectomy [removal of the large intestine], or who have had a colectomy and now have a pouch of small intestine connected to their rectum [a J-pouch])
- The American Gastroenterological Association: www.gastro.org

Your library and local bookstore can be sources of good information, too. We recommend asking your doctors about appropriate books if your child has IBD. Hospital patient libraries often have books and videotapes as well.

For information on insurance appeals, family medical leave, and school advocacy, an excellent Web site is www.advocacyforpatients. org. The organization Advocacy for Patients with Chronic Illness is headed by Jennifer Jaff, an attorney with special expertise in the coverage of issues facing patients with inflammatory bowel disease.

This is a busy time in the field of inflammatory bowel disease. New information on causes and treatments is changing daily, so it is important to keep informed. The information sources above will expand your knowledge of IBD. You should remember, however, that no two IBD patients are alike. Individual help and advice is as close as your telephone—take advantage of your doctor's knowledge.

Frequently Asked Questions

What is inflammatory bowel disease?

Inflammatory bowel disease (IBD) is a general name for two different conditions: Crohn disease (CD) and ulcerative colitis (UC). CD and UC cause damage to different parts of the digestive (gastrointestinal, or GI) tract and sometimes to other parts of the body as well.

What is Crohn disease?

Crohn disease is an ongoing disease that causes inflammation (swelling and irritation) of the digestive tract. Although it can involve any area of the GI tract from the mouth to the anus, it most commonly affects the small intestine, colon (large intestine), or both.

Why is my condition called Crohn disease?

The disease is named after Dr. Burrill Crohn. In 1932, Dr. Crohn and two colleagues, Dr. Leon Ginzburg and Dr. Gordon Oppenheimer, published the first paper describing what is now known as Crohn disease.

What is ulcerative colitis (UC)?

UC an ongoing disease that causes inflammation (swelling and irritation) of the digestive tract. Unlike Crohn disease, UC only causes inflammation of the colon (large intestine).

How long have I had my IBD?

No one knows for sure. Some people have years of symptoms before the diagnosis is made, while in others the symptoms appear suddenly. Both groups may have had intestinal inflammation for days, months, or years, even though they didn't experience any symptoms at all for most of that time.

Will I have to live with IBD for the rest of my life?

As this book goes to print, both Crohn disease and ulcerative colitis are considered chronic illnesses, which means that you will have the disease for the rest of your life. Medication can reduce the inflammation that is causing symptoms. When inflammation is reduced, the tissue can heal and you can achieve remission (disappearance of any signs of disease).

Is there a cure for Crohn disease or ulcerative colitis?

At this time, there is no medical or surgical cure for Crohn disease. Ulcerative colitis can be cured with surgery.

How will IBD affect my day-to-day life?

The goal of your healthcare team is to allow your day-to-day life to continue without interruption. You should be able to attend school and activities outside school, go to work, and have a normal life.

Is this disease going to change what I can or can't eat or drink?

Changes in your diet may be necessary to relieve symptoms such as stomach pain or loose bowel movements (diarrhea). Discuss your diet with the doctors and nurses who help take care of you. Foods affect each of us differently, so it is important to pay attention to what foods bother your stomach and avoid them in the future.

I play sports. Will IBD affect my ability to play?

No. Playing sports is important for bone development. There are many professional athletes with IBD. Crohn disease, however, as well as some medications such as steroids, when taken for many months, can weaken the bones. Your doctor may want you to have a DEXA scan (an x-ray measure of bone strength) before you begin playing contact sports such as football or soccer.

Will IBD affect my social life?

We hope that having IBD will not affect your social life. It is up to you to decide whether you tell your friends about your illness. It is always helpful to have allies who can help if should you need it.

How did I get IBD in the first place?

We still don't know the cause of either form of IBD. Development of this disease is surely a complex process involving genetics, the immune system, and something in the environment. According to the current theory, the genes you inherited are vulnerable to something in the environment. This environmental factor acts as a trigger, causing your immune system to attack the digestive tract. Once the immune system is switched on, it does not recognize the signal to turn off the attack at the correct time. This results in ongoing tissue damage and causes the symptoms of IBD.

Did I do something to cause this?

The answer is a resounding *no*. Your actions did not cause this disease.

Where can I find out more information?

The North American Society for Pediatric Gastroenterology, Hepatology, and Nutrition hosts a Web site at www.naspghan.org, which provides information for children and adolescents with IBD and their parents. NASPGHAN and the Children's Digestive Health and Nutrition Foundation (CDHNF) cosponsor a Web site for children with IBD, their parents, and their health care providers. The site can be found at www.kidsibd.org.

The Crohn's and Colitis Foundation of America hosts a Web site for children and adolescents and provides pamphlets and books on the subject. For the Crohn's and Colitis Foundation, visit www.ccfa.org; the teen site can be found at www.ucandcrohns.org.

See chapter 22 for additional helpful Web sites. (Remember: the Internet is a useful resource, but read with caution—not all of the information available is based in fact.)

Are there many other people who have IBD?

It is estimated that approximately 1 million Americans have inflammatory bowel disease. It occurs in people of all ages. Both Crohn disease and ulcerative colitis commonly develop in teenagers and young adults. Ten percent of those affected by IBD are under 18 years of age (100,000 people in the United States).

How will my life change because I have this disease?

You will probably need to take medication daily. You will have more doctor's appointments than before. You may need to stay in the hospital at some point.

Can this disease trigger any other health problems?

A number of other problems are, at times, associated with IBD. These can include eye problems, liver problems, kidney stones, mouth ulcers, fevers, sores around your bottom, joint problems, and skin problems.

Do I have to have surgery?

Medication is the main treatment for patients with IBD. However, some patients will require surgery over time. There is a place for surgery in treating Crohn disease and ulcerative colitis. Surgery may be necessary in Crohn disease to remove very narrowed areas of intestine (strictures) that can cause blockages, or areas of severe disease that do not respond to treatments. It may also be necessary to remove fistulas—abnormal connections between loops of intestines or between intestines and other organs—or to drain abscesses (pockets of pus), if they develop.

In ulcerative colitis, surgery to remove the large intestine will eliminate or cure the disease. Surgery can be considered if severe symptoms do not respond to medical treatments, or if serious complications develop.

Do I have to be hooked up to any equipment?

Most people do not need any special equipment.

How do you treat IBD?

IBD is treated with medications, dietary changes, and, in some cases, surgery.

Is this disease genetic? Am I going to pass it on to my kids?

Genetics research has discovered several genes associated with Crohn disease and ulcerative colitis. We know that some families have several members with IBD, but some patients have no family history. There is a genetic link, but it remains unclear as to what it means at this point. Children born to parents who have IBD have a slightly increased risk of developing IBD, but this risk is small.

Will IBD cause me pain?

Abdominal pain, rectal pain, and joint pain are symptoms associated with IBD. These symptoms can usually be controlled by the medications and other treatments prescribed by your doctor.

What are the symptoms of IBD?

Diarrhea, weight loss, and abdominal pain are the most common symptoms for children with Crohn disease. Blood in the stool, lack of appetite, fevers, joint pain, sores on the skin, and redness of the whites of the eye are less common symptoms. Some children also have trouble gaining weight and growing, even when they do not have many other obvious symptoms.

Ulcerative colitis usually causes crampy abdominal pain and bloody diarrhea. Decreased appetite and weight loss occur when the illness is active, but poor growth in height is rare.

Will the medications make me feel different?

Most medications improve patients' symptoms and make them feel better. However, medications can, at times, cause side effects. For example, prednisone (a steroid) may make you moody—down on some days, happy on others. It will also make you very hungry. Methotrexate (a medicine that modifies the immune system) may cause nausea the day after you take it. Mesalamine (an anti-inflammatory) may cause headaches, which will disappear when the dose of the medication is reduced.

Is my IBD going to get worse or better over time?

Both Crohn disease and ulcerative colitis have periods of quiet (remission), when you feel fine, and periods of activity (flareups), when your symptoms are active. It is impossible to predict how you will feel, but the goals of your treatment are to decrease the inflammation, heal the damaged tissue, and make you feel well, giving you the best quality of life possible.

Can I take care of my condition by myself, or do I need my mother, father, or guardian to help?

Younger children need their parents to make sure they are taking their medicines and eating well. As you get older, you will need to be responsible for your medications and for taking good care of yourself in general. This includes getting enough sleep and eating well. You will be able to lead an independent and productive life on your own when the time comes.

What's going to happen if I do eat or drink something that I shouldn't?

Different people react differently, but in general, you might get abdominal pain or loose bowel movements.

How bad is my case in comparison to other people who have this condition?

Everyone is different. It is best not to compare yourself to others.

How often will I feel fine, compared to the times I am in pain or uncomfortable?

There is no way to predict how you will feel. With appropriate treatment, we hope that you will feel well most of the time.

This whole endoscopy thing doesn't sound very appealing. Is it really necessary that I do this, and if so, how often?

A colonoscopy (endoscopic examination of the colon) is necessary to make the diagnosis of Crohn disease and ulcerative colitis. An upper endoscopy is needed when you have symptoms that suggest inflammation in your esophagus (food pipe), stomach, or small intestine. You will need these tests when the doctor is first finding out why you have been feeling bad. After you have started treatments, there may be circumstances when you will need to have the tests again, to help the doctor understand how your treatments are working. There is no fixed schedule for these tests, but after you have been ill for eight or nine years, you will probably need to undergo a colonoscopy every few years to make sure no complications are developing.

Will I need any other uncomfortable tests or treatments?

An upper GI series (an x-ray where you have to drink barium) is usually necessary to make a picture of the intestines and show the doctor whether there is inflammation. There may also be other tests that are uncomfortable. These will be explained to you at the time you need them so that you know what to expect.

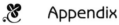 **Appendix**
A Guide to IBD Medications by Trade Name, Generic Name, and Medication Class

Adapted from *NASPGHAN Personal IBD Notebook*

Common IBD Medications (by trade name)

Trade name	Generic name	Dosage forms	Medication class
Anusol-HC ointment	Hydrocortisone	Ointment (1%, 2.5%)	Corticosteroid
Anusol-HC suppository	Hydrocortisone	Suppository (25 mg)	Corticosteroid
Asacol	Mesalamine	Tablet (400 mg)	5-ASA
Azasan	Azathioprine	Tablet (25, 50, 75 mg)	Immunomodulator
Azulfidine	Sulfasalazine	Tablet (500 mg)	5-ASA
Canasa	Mesalamine	Suppository (500 mg, 1 gm)	5-ASA
Cipro	Ciprofloxacin	Capsule (250 mg)	Antibiotic
Colazal	Balsalazide	Capsule (750 mg)	5-ASA
Cortenema	Hydrocortisone	Enema (100 mg/60 mL)	Corticosteroid
Cortifoam	Hydrocortisone	Rectal foam (10%)	Corticosteroid
Deltasone	Prednisone	Tablet (2.5, 5, 10, 20 mg)	Corticosteroid
Dipentum	Olsalazine	Tablet (250 mg)	5-ASA
Entocort EC	Budesonide	Capsule (3mg)	Corticosteroid
Flagyl	Metronidazole	Tablet (250, 500 mg) Capsule (375 mg)	Antibiotic
Folex	Methotrexate	Tablet (2.5 mg) Injection (25 mg/mL)	Immunomodulator
Humira	Adalimumab	Injection (40 mg syringe)	Biological agent
Imuran	Azathioprine	Tablet (50 mg)	Immunomodulator

Common IBD Medications (by trade name) *(continued)*

Trade name	Generic name	Dosage forms	Medication class
Medrol	Methyl-prednisolone	Tablet (2, 4, 8, 16, 32 mg)	Corticosteroid
Mercaptopurine	6-Mercaptopurine	Tablet (50 mg)	Immunomodulator
Mexate	Methotrexate	Tablet (2.5 mg) Injection (25 mg/mL)	Immunomodulator
Neoral	Cyclosporine	Capsule (25, 100 mg) Liquid (100 mg/mL)	Immunomodulator
Pediapred	Prednisolone	Liquid (5 mg/5 mL)	Corticosteroid
Pentasa	Mesalamine	Capsule (250, 500 mg)	5-ASA
Prelone	Prednisolone	Liquid (15 mg/5 mL)	Corticosteroid
Prevacid	Lansoprazole	Capsule (15, 30 mg) Liquid (1 mg/mL)	Acid blocker
Prilosec	Omeprazole	Capsule (10, 20 mg)	Acid blocker
ProctoFoam-HC	Hydrocortisone	Rectal foam (1%)	Corticosteroid
Purinethol	Mercaptopurine	Tablet (50 mg)	Immunomodulator
Remicade	Infliximab	Injection (100 mg)	Biological agent
Rheumatrex	Methotrexate	Tablet (2.5 mg) Injection (25 mg/mL)	Immunomodulator
Rowasa	Mesalamine	Enema (1 gram)	5-ASA
Xifaxin	Rifaximin	Tablet (200 mg)	Antibiotic
Zantac	Ranitidine	Tablet (150 mg) Liquid (15 mg/mL)	Acid blocker

Common IBD Medications (by generic name)

Generic name	Trade name	Dosage forms	Medication class
6-Mercaptopurine	Purinethol, Mercaptopurine	Tablet (50 mg)	Immunomodulator
Adalimumab	Humira	Injection (40 mg syringe)	Biological agent
Azathioprine	Imuran, Azasan	Tablet (25, 50, 75 mg)	Immunomodulator
Balsalazide	Colazal	Capsule (750 mg)	5-ASA

Generic name	Trade name	Dosage forms	Medication class
Budesonide	Entocort EC	Capsule (3 mg)	Corticosteroid
Ciprofloxacin	Cipro	Capsule (250 mg)	Antibiotic
Cyclosporine	Neoral	Capsule (25, 100 mg) Liquid (100 mg/mL)	Immunomodulator
Hydrocortisone	Anusol-HC ointment	Ointment (1%, 2.5%)	Corticosteroid
Hydrocortisone	Anusol-HC suppository	Suppository (25 mg)	Corticosteroid
Hydrocortisone	Cortenema	Enema (100 mg/60 mL)	Corticosteroid
Hydrocortisone	Cortifoam	Rectal foam (10%)	Corticosteroid
Hydrocortisone	ProctoFoam-HC	Rectal foam (1%)	Corticosteroid
Infliximab	Remicade	Injection (100 mg)	Biological agent
Lansoprazole	Prevacid	Capsule (15, 30 mg) Liquid (1 mg/mL)	Acid blocker
Mesalamine	Asacol	Tablet (400 mg)	5-ASA
Mesalamine	Canasa	Suppository (500 mg, 1 gm)	5-ASA
Mesalamine	Pentasa	Capsule (250, 500 mg)	5-ASA
Mesalamine	Rowasa	Enema (1 gram)	5-ASA
Methotrexate	Folex	Tablet (2.5 mg) Injection (25 mg/mL)	Immunomodulator
Methotrexate	Mexate	Tablet (2.5 mg) Injection (25 mg/mL)	Immunomodulator
Methotrexate	Rheumatrex	Tablet (2.5 mg) Injection (25 mg/mL)	Immunomodulator
Methyl-prednisolone	Medrol	Tablet (2, 4, 8, 16, 32 mg)	Corticosteroid
Metronidazole	Flagyl	Tablet (250, 500 mg) Capsule (375 mg)	Antibiotic
Olsalazine	Dipentum	Tablet (250 mg)	5-ASA
Omeprazole	Prilosec	Capsule (10, 20 mg)	Acid blocker

Common IBD Medications (by generic name) *(continued)*

Generic name	Trade name	Dosage forms	Medication class
Prednisolone	Pediapred	Liquid (5 mg/5 mL)	Corticosteroid
Prednisolone	Prelone	Liquid (15 mg/5 mL)	Corticosteroid
Prednisone	Deltasone	Tablet (2.5, 5, 10, 20 mg)	Corticosteroid
Ranitidine	Zantac	Tablet (150 mg) Liquid (15 mg/mL)	Acid blocker
Rifaximin	Xifaxin	Tablet (200 mg)	Antibiotic
Sulfasalazine	Azulfidine	Tablet (500 mg)	5-ASA

Common IBD Medications (by medication class)

Medication class	Trade name	Generic name	Dosage forms
5-ASA	Asacol	Mesalamine	Tablet (400 mg)
5-ASA	Azulfidine	Sulfasalazine	Tablet (500 mg)
5-ASA	Canasa	Mesalamine	Suppository (500 mg, 1 gm)
5-ASA	Colazal	Balsalazide	Capsule (750 mg)
5-ASA	Dipentum	Olsalazine	Tablet (250 mg)
5-ASA	Pentasa	Mesalamine	Capsule (250, 500 mg)
5-ASA	Rowasa	Mesalamine	Enema (1 gram)
Acid blocker	Prevacid	Lansoprazole	Capsule (15, 30 mg) Liquid (1 mg/mL)
Acid blocker	Prilosec	Omeprazole	Capsule (10, 20 mg)
Acid blocker	Zantac	Ranitidine	Tablet (150 mg) Liquid (15 mg/mL)
Antibiotic	Cipro	Ciprofloxacin	Capsule (250 mg)
Antibiotic	Flagyl	Metronidazole	Tablet (250 mg)
Antibiotic	Xifaxin	Rifaximin	Tablet (200 mg)
Biological agent	Humira	Adalimumab	Injection (40 mg syringe)
Biological agent	Remicade	Infliximab	Injection (100 mg)

Medication class	Trade name	Generic name	Dosage forms
Corticosteroid	Anusol-HC ointment	Hydrocortisone	Ointment (1%, 2.5%)
Corticosteroid	Anusol-HC suppository	Hydrocortisone	Suppository (25 mg)
Corticosteroid	Cortenema	Hydrocortisone	Enema (100 mg/60 mL)
Corticosteroid	Cortifoam	Hydrocortisone	Rectal foam (10%)
Corticosteroid	Deltasone	Prednisone	Tablet (2.5, 5, 10, 20 mg)
Corticosteroid	Entocort EC	Budesonide	Capsule (3 mg)
Corticosteroid	Medrol	Methyl-prednisolone	Tablet (2, 4, 8, 16, 32 mg)
Corticosteroid	Pediapred	Prednisolone	Liquid (5 mg/5 mL)
Corticosteroid	Prelone	Prednisolone	Liquid (15 mg/5 mL)
Corticosteroid	ProctoFoam-HC	Hydrocortisone	Rectal foam (1%)
Immunomodulator	Folex	Methotrexate	Tablet (2.5 mg) Injection (25 mg/mL)
Immunomodulator	Imuran, Azasan	Azathioprine	Tablet (25, 50, 75 mg)
Immunomodulator	Mexate	Methotrexate	Tablet (2.5 mg) Injection (25 mg/mL)
Immunomodulator	Neoral	Cyclosporine	Capsule (25, 100 mg) Liquid (100 mg/mL)
Immunomodulator	Purinethol, Mercaptopurine	6-Mercaptopurine	Tablet (50 mg)
Immunomodulator	Rheumatrex	Methotrexate	Tablet (2.5 mg) Injection (25 mg/mL)

❧ Glossary

Below are common terms and abbreviations you might see or hear at the doctor's office or the hospital. *Italicized* words in the definition are also defined in this glossary.

Abscess: A "pocket" of pus in the body, caused by infection

Albumin: A protein that is measured in blood tests; albumin level is a good indicator of inflammation, and low levels mean increased inflammation

Anastomosis: The process of surgically joining two hollow organs, often after the tissue originally joining them has been surgically removed (*resected*)

Anemia: Lower than normal amounts of *hemoglobin* in the red cells of the blood

Ankylosing spondylitis: A form of joint inflammation primarily involving the spine and the lower back, sometimes seen in patients with IBD

Antibody tests: Blood tests that are sometimes used by physicians to suggest if a patient may have Crohn disease or colitis; these tests are not considered definitive in making a diagnosis of IBD and are not a substitute for x-rays and endoscopy

Anus: The opening through which stool (a bowel movement) leaves the body

Arthralgia: Pains in the joints, frequently felt by persons with IBD

Arthritis: Inflammation (swelling) of a joint, accompanied by pain, heat, or redness

5-ASA (5-aminosalicylic acid): Another name for the active component of *mesalamine*, olsalazine, balsalazide, and sulfasalazine

Aseptic necrosis: A complication of the long-term use of high-dose steroids, in which a joint (usually the hip) goes through massive destruction

Autoimmunity: An inflammatory reaction to one's own tissues

Barium: A white, chalky substance, which helps show parts of the *GI tract* on an x-ray

Barium enema: An x-ray exam of the *colon* and *rectum*, after liquid *barium* has been given to the patient through the *anus*

BE: Abbreviation for *barium enema*

BID: Abbreviation for twice a day (Latin: *bis in die*)

Biopsy: A small piece of tissue taken from an area of the body and checked under a microscope

BP: Abbreviation for blood pressure

C&S: Abbreviation for culture and sensitivity, a test for bacteria in blood and urine samples

CAT Scan: See *CT scan*

CBC: Abbreviation for complete blood count, a type of blood test

CD: Abbreviation for *Crohn disease*

Celiac disease: An intolerance to gluten, a protein found in rye, barley, and oats; celiac disease causes inflammation of the small intestine, and the symptoms can mimic those of Crohn disease

Colectomy: Removal of part or all of the *colon*

Colitis: Inflammation of the large intestine

Colon: The large intestine

Colonoscopy: A test in which a flexible, lighted tube is inserted through the *rectum* to examine the large intestine

Colostomy: An opening, created through surgery, that connects the large intestine to the outside of the body through the skin of the abdomen (belly area); stool leaves the body through this opening into a special bag, called an appliance

Comprehensive metabolic panel (CMP): Twelve blood tests that are run from a single blood sample, so that only one blood draw is needed

C-reactive protein (CRP): A blood test that measures inflammation; this protein may be elevated in cases of active IBD

Crohn disease: A chronic disease that causes inflammation of the small intestine, large intestine, or both

CT scan: Abbreviation for computed tomography scan, a special type of x-ray

CXR: Abbreviation for chest x-ray

Cytokine: A protein released by cells of the immune system that helps cells "talk" to one another

Digestive tract: The *gastrointestinal tract*

Discharge summary: A summary, dictated by the physician during or after a patient's hospital stay, which includes any tests or operations performed, laboratory data, the patient's condition when they leave the hospital, and plans for follow-up care

Distal: Away from the center or away from the beginning; in the *GI tract*, a distal point would be close to the *anus*

Distension: An uncomfortable swelling in the abdomen, often caused by excessive amounts of gas and fluids in the intestine

Dx: Abbreviation for diagnosis

Dysplasia: Changes in cells that may predict the development of cancer

E. nodosum: Abbreviation for *erythema nodosum*, a skin rash

ECG (EKG): Abbreviation for electrocardiogram, the measurement of the electrical activity of the heart

Edema: Accumulation of too much fluids in the tissues, resulting in swelling

Electrolytes: Chemicals, such as salts, that are necessary for the body to keep working

Elemental diet: A specially prepared liquid meal that does not contain any foods to which people will normally have a reaction

Endoscopy: The examination of the inside of a hollow organ, such as the bowel, using special lighted tubes

Enteral nutrition: Delivering food and nutrients into the stomach and intestine, often using a *nasogastric tube*

Enterocyte: Absorptive cell in the *intestinal epithelium*

Episcleritis: Inflammation of the eye, sometimes seen in patients with IBD

Erythema nodosum: Reddish purple swellings, occasionally seen on the lower legs during flareups of Crohn disease and ulcerative colitis

ESR: Abbreviation for erythrocyte sedimentation rate, a type of blood test that can point to an inflammatory condition in the body

Exacerbation: A worsening of symptoms; a relapse; a flareup; a period of active disease

Excision: Surgical removal

Extraintestinal manifestations: Inflammation of other organ systems (skin, joints, eye) sometimes seen in patients with IBD

Exudate: A whitish material seen in an inflamed colon, usually consisting of mucus and white blood cells (pus)

Febrile: Running a fever

Fissure: A crack in the skin; with Crohn disease, usually near the area of the *anus*

Fistula: An abnormal connection between two locations in the body; for example, the connection can be between loops of intestine, or between the intestine and another structure, such as the bladder, vagina, or skin

Folic acid: One of the vitamins responsible for the maintenance of red blood cells

Fulminant: Disease that develops extremely quickly

Gastroenterologist: A physician specially trained in the diagnosis and treatment of patients with stomach and intestinal disease

Gastroesophageal reflux (GER): The regurgitation of stomach acid and food back into the esophagus, often causing heartburn or vomiting

Gastrointestinal tract (GI tract): The digestive system, extending from the stomach to the *anus* and including the small and large intestine

GI: Abbreviation for *gastrointestinal* (meaning stomach and intestines)

GI tract: Abbreviation for *gastrointestinal tract*

Granuloma: A characteristic inflammatory reaction that can be seen in about 30% of Crohn disease patients

Gut: General word for intestine or bowel

H&P: Abbreviation for *history and physical examination*

Hct: Abbreviation for *hematocrit*

Hematocrit: A measure of the number of red blood cells in whole blood; patients with *anemia* have low levels of hematocrit

Hemoglobin: The part of red blood cells that carries oxygen; low levels of hemoglobin result in *anemia*

Hemorrhage: Abnormally heavy bleeding

Hemorrhoids: Painful, enlarged veins of the lower *rectum* and *anus*, sometimes seen as a complication in people with IBD

Hgb: Abbreviation for *hemoglobin*

History and physical examination: A record that contains a person's complete medical history, as well as results from physical exams

HPI: Abbreviation for history of present illness

Hygiene hypothesis: The theory that growing up in a cleaner environment with fewer infections may increase the risk of autoimmune disease like diabetes and IBD

Hyperalimentation: A way of giving patients additional nutrition (food) through a vein, if they cannot get all their body's dietary needs through eating; also known as total parenteral nutrition (TPN)

IBD: Abbreviation for *inflammatory bowel disease*

IBS: Abbreviation for *irritable bowel syndrome*

Idiopathic: Of unknown cause

Ileitis: Inflammation of the lower part of the small intestine, seen commonly in Crohn disease

Ileoanal anastomosis: A newer operation (also known as the pull-through) for ulcerative colitis, in which an internal pouch is created after a *colectomy*; because the *rectum* is not removed, the patient continues to pass stool through the *anus*

Ileocecal valve: The border between the end of the small intestine and the beginning of the large intestine

Ileostomy: An opening, created through surgery, that connects the *ileum* to the outside of the body through the skin of the abdomen (belly area); stool leaves the body through this opening into a special bag, called an appliance

Ileum: The lower third of the small intestine, closest to the *colon*

Ileus: Temporary paralysis of the bowel, often resulting from surgery, abdominal infection, or *electrolyte* imbalance

IM: Abbreviation for intramuscular, meaning into a muscle

Immunology: Study of the body's immune response to disease

Immunomodulators: Drugs that suppress (hold back) or strengthen the body's immune response

Incontinence: In IBD, the inability to keep stool in the body (resulting in accidents), usually because the *rectum* is inflamed

Indeterminate colitis: A form of IBD with features of both ulcerative colitis and Crohn disease

Induction treatment: Using strong medications to treat a flare and get a sick patient well

Inflammatory bowel disease: A collective term for Crohn disease and ulcerative colitis

Intestinal epithelium: Lining of the small intestine

Intractable: Isn't helped by medical treatments

Irritable bowel syndrome: Abdominal discomfort, sometimes mistakenly called "spastic colitis"; this condition does not cause inflammation of the *colon* and has no relationship to IBD

IV: Abbreviation for intravenous, meaning into a vein

KUB: Kidneys-ureter-bladder

Lactose breath test: A test that involves drinking a liquid rich in milk sugar; breath samples are then taken over a period to determine whether there is enough lactase (an enzyme that breaks down milk sugar) in the body

Lactose intolerance (or lactase deficiency): A condition caused by a decrease or absence of the enzyme lactase, which aids in the breakdown of lactose (milk sugar)

Laparoscopy: Surgical procedure in which instruments are inserted into the abdomen through several small openings, leaving several very small scars

Laparotomy (or open surgery): A surgery requiring one large abdominal incision

Left-sided colitis: A form of ulcerative colitis where only a portion of the colon (the rectum, sigmoid, and descending colon) is inflamed

Leukocytosis: An increased number of white blood cells in circulation; a sign of infection

Lumen (intestinal): The hollow area inside the intestine where food and liquid pass through

Magnetic resonance imaging (MRI): An imaging study using magnets to show the appearance of organs inside the body

Maintenance therapies (or maintenance treatment): Medications taken when a patient with IBD has the disease under control, to prevent flares

Mesalamine: The generic name for 5-ASA, a drug used to treat inflamed intestine with few, if any, side effects

Motility: In the digestive tract, movement of the muscles that propel food through the intestines

MRI: Abbreviation for *magnetic resonance imaging*

Mucus: In the digestive tract, a clear or whitish substance produced by the intestine, which may be found in the stool

Nasogastric tube (NG tube): A thin, flexible tube passed through the nose or the mouth; an NG tube is used to remove liquids and air that collect in the stomach, when the bowel is obstructed or after intestinal surgery; it is also used to deliver nutrients (food) into the stomach

NPO: Abbreviation for nothing by mouth (Latin: *nihil per os*)

Obstruction: In the digestive tract, a blockage of the small or large intestine that prevents the normal passage of intestinal contents

Occult blood: Invisible blood in the stool, often an indication of disease activity; simple lab tests can determine the presence of occult blood

Operative report: A complete record of an operation, dictated by the surgeon after surgery

Ostomy: An artificial opening made through surgery

Pancolitis: Ulcerative colitis that involves the entire large intestine; this is the type of ulcerative colitis that is most common in children

Parenteral nutrition (PN): A way of providing nutrition to people who cannot take enough food into their stomach or intestines; in a person receiving PN, nutrients (including carbohydrates, fat, and proteins) are delivered directly into a vein

Pathogen: A bacterium or virus that causes disease

Pathogenesis: The origin and development of disease

Pathology report: Results of examination of any tissues removed from the body during surgery or *biopsy*

Peptic ulcers: Erosions in the lining of the stomach or duodenum (first part of the small intestine)

Percutaneous endoscopic gastrostomy (PEG): Using an endoscope to place a feeding tube into the stomach

Perforation: The development of a hole in an organ; in the digestive tract, a perforation is usually a hole in the bowel wall, allowing what is inside the intestines to spill into the abdominal cavity

Perianal: The area around the anal opening; this area may become inflamed and irritated in persons with IBD

Peristalsis: The normal regular movements of the stomach and intestines

Peristomal: The area immediately surrounding the *stoma*

Peritonitis: Inflammation of the peritoneum (the membrane enclosing the abdominal organs); peritonitis usually results from an intestinal *perforation* or infection

Pharynx: Throat

Plt: Abbreviation for platelet count

PO: Abbreviation for by mouth (Latin: *per os*)

Polygenic: Caused by multiple inherited genes

Polyp: A small growth in the intestine; these can cause rectal bleeding in young children, but they are almost never cancerous

Pouchitis: Inflammation of the ileoanal pouch (a pouch created by a surgical procedure performed in patients with ulcerative colitis)

Primary sclerosing cholangitis (PSC): An autoimmune disease that causes scarring of the bile ducts, leading to fatigue and jaundice (yellow skin). This disease is seen in 2 to 4 percent of patients with Crohn or colitis

Proctectomy: Surgical removal of the *rectum*

Proctitis: Inflammation of the *rectum*

Proctocolectomy: Removal of the entire *colon* and *rectum*

Progress notes: A daily record of a patient's progress, test results, and so forth, completed by the professionals who care for the patient

Prolapse: The falling, or protrusion (pushing forward), of an organ

PRN: Abbreviation for as needed (Latin: *pro re nata*)

Proximal: Closer to the beginning; in the digestive tract, a proximal point is closer to the mouth

PSC: Abbreviation for primary sclerosing cholangitis

Pyoderma gangrenosum: A type of sore or ulcer that sometimes occurs on the arms or legs of persons with IBD

Q4H: Abbreviation for every four hours

QD: Abbreviation for every day

QID: Abbreviation for four times per day

QOD: Abbreviation for every other day

RAP: Abbreviation for recurrent abdominal pain

RBC: Abbreviation for *red blood cell*

Rectum: The part of the intestine that connects the *colon* to the *anus*

Regional enteritis: A name for Crohn disease affecting the small intestine

Remission: A lessening of symptoms and a return to good health

Resection: Surgical removal

Reservoir: A surgically created pouch that collects waste

RX: Abbreviation for medications

S: Abbreviation for without (Latin: *sans*)

Sacroiliitis: Inflammation of the large joints where the spine meets the pelvis in the lower back

SBFT: Abbreviation for small bowel follow-through, used when describing an upper GI x-ray in which *barium* is followed all the way through the entire small intestine (see also *upper GI series*)

SED Rate: See ESR

Sedimentation rate: A blood test that measures inflammation; in active Crohn disease and ulcerative colitis, the sedimentation rate may be increased

Short bowel syndrome: A condition in which so much diseased bowel has been surgically removed that the remaining intestine can no longer absorb sufficient nutrients

Sigmoidoscopy: A test in which a lighted tube is passed through the *rectum* into the part of the *colon* nearest to it

Small bowel: Small intestine

Spastic colon: An old, obsolete term sometimes used to describe irritable bowel syndrome

Sphincter: A ring of muscle tissue keeping certain parts of the digestive tract (like the *anus*) closed

Stenosis: A narrowing of an area

Stoma: A surgically created opening of the bowel through the skin in the abdomen

Stricture: Narrowing; in IBD, a narrowed area of intestine caused by active inflammation or scar tissue

Strictureplasty: A surgical procedure that widens narrowed areas of intestine (*strictures*)

Subtotal colectomy: Removal of part or most of the *colon*, leaving a part (usually the *rectum*) intact

Sutures: Materials used in surgery to close wounds

Tenesmus: A constant urge to empty the bowel (pass stool), usually caused by inflammation of the *rectum*

TID: Abbreviation for three times a day

Total parenteral nutrition (TPN): See *hyperalimentation*

Toxic megacolon: Severe dilation (enlargement) of the colon in ulcerative colitis (or occasionally in Crohn disease), which may lead to *perforation*

TPR: Abbreviation for temperature, pulse, and respiration

Transmural inflammation: Inflammation involving the whole thickness of the intestinal wall, seen in Crohn's but not ulcerative colitis

Tx: Abbreviation for *treatment*

Ulcerative colitis: A chronic disease that causes inflammation of the large intestine

Ulcerative proctitis: A form of ulcerative colitis where only the rectum is inflamed

Ultrasound: An imaging study using sound waves to show the appearance of organs inside the body

Upper endoscopy (esophagogastroduodenoscopy, EGD): An examination where a gastroenterologist examines the esophagus, stomach, and duodenum with a camera

Upper GI series (UGI): An x-ray exam of the esophagus, stomach, and duodenum (first part of the small intestine) performed in a fasting patient after he or she drinks liquid *barium*; the exam can be made longer to allow the barium to go through the entire small intestine. The x-ray is then known as an upper GI series with small bowel follow-through (see *SBFT*)

US or U/S: Abbreviation for *ultrasound*

Uveitis: Inflammation of the eye sometimes seen in IBD

Villi: Fingerlike projections of absorptive cells that line the intestine and help in the digestion and absorption of food

WBC: Abbreviation for *white blood cell*

Within normal limits: A term used to describe a laboratory test result that is similar to that seen in healthy people

WNL: Abbreviation for *within normal limits*

X-ray reports: Results of x-ray studies (tests)

Index

About the North American Society for Pediatric Gastroenterology, Hepatology and Nutrition (NASPGHAN) and the Children's Digestive Health and Nutrition Foundation (CDHNF)

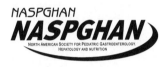

Mission

The mission of the North American Society for Pediatric Gastroenterology, Hepatology and Nutrition is to advance understanding of normal development, physiology, and pathophysiology of diseases of the gastrointestinal tract and liver in children, improve quality of care by fostering the dissemination of this knowledge through scientific meetings, professional and public education, and policy development, and serve as an effective voice for members and the profession.

The membership of NASPGHAN consists of more than 1500 pediatric gastroenterologists, predominantly in 46 states, the District of Columbia, Puerto Rico, Mexico, and 8 provinces in Canada.

NASPGHAN strives to improve the care of infants, children, and adolescents with digestive disorders by promoting advances in clinical care, research, and education. Pediatric gastroenterologists specialize in the care of children with chronic abdominal pain, diarrhea, constipation, vomiting, bleeding from the GI tract, inflammatory bowel disease, liver diseases, diseases of the pancreas, poor weight gain, and nutritional problems.

Pediatric gastroenterologists specialize in gastroesophageal reflux (GER), peptic ulcers, *H. pylori*, celiac disease, Crohn's disease, ulcerative colitis, Hirschsprung's disease, cyclic vomiting, polyps, gallstones, hepatitis, biliary atresia, jaundice, pancreatitis, lactose malabsorption, failure to thrive, and other common and rare disorders. Most pediatric gastroenterologists perform endoscopy, colonoscopy, esophageal pH probe studies, esophageal and rectal manometry, and liver biopsies.

Objectives

NASPGHAN's objectives include but are not limited to:

Improving the digestive health and nutrition of children worldwide and particularly in North America.

Fostering dialogue and research on pertinent issues that impact the pediatric gastroenterology patient and their family.

Providing opportunities for clinicians and researchers to gain knowledge of the scientific advances in the field of pediatric gastroenterology.

Disseminating the wealth of scientific information that exists in order to improve clinical outcomes and advance the practice of pediatric gastroenterology and nutrition.

CDHNF

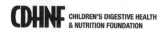 CHILDREN'S DIGESTIVE HEALTH & NUTRITION FOUNDATION

Mission

To fund and promote research and educational programs that will advance the creation, application, and dissemination of knowledge of gastrointestinal, hepatobiliary, pancreatic, and nutritional disorders in children.

To identify, encourage, support, and coordinate scientific research and professional study of these pediatric disorders.

To strengthen the role of pediatric gastrointestinal and nutritional scientists as leaders in research and education in these medical and health care fields.

To evaluate and improve the quality and availability of medical care for children with digestive disorders.

To support the research and educational programs of NASPGHAN.

Objective

The Children's Digestive Health and Nutrition Foundation (CDHNF) has a single goal: to improve the treatment and management of gastrointestinal, hepatobiliary, pancreatic, and nutritional disorders in children. Through our work, we provide information and resources to parents, patients, and medical professionals dealing with these disorders.

CDHNF was founded by the North American Society for Pediatric Gastroenterology, Hepatology and Nutrition (NASPGHAN). CDHNF promotes research, education, and awareness of pediatric digestive and nutritional disorders.

Library of Congress Cataloging-in-Publication Data

Your child with inflammatory bowel disease: a family guide for caregiving /
North American Society for Pediatric Gastroenterology, Hepatology and
Nutrition ; editors-in-chief Maria Oliva-Hemker, David Ziring,
Athos Bousvaros.
    p.   cm.
    Includes index.
    ISBN-13: 978-0-8018-9555-5 (hardcover: alk. paper)
    ISBN-10: 0-8018-9555-3 (hardcover: alk. paper)
    ISBN-13: 978-0-8018-9556-2 (pbk.: alk. paper)
    ISBN-10: 0-8018-9556-1 (pbk.: alk. paper)
    1. Inflammatory bowel diseases—Popular works. 2. Gastroenteritis
in children—Popular works. 3. Caregivers—Popular works.
I. Oliva-Hemker, Maria. II. Ziring, David. III. Bousvaros, Athos.
IV. North American Society for Pediatric Gastroenterology,
Hepatology and Nutrition.
    RJ456.G3Y68 2010
    618.92′344—dc22   2009037372

A catalog record for this book is available from the British Library.